DO YOU KNOW YOUR
MEDICAL CONDITIONS
?

From

Abortion to Zoster

Compiled by

DR. TERRY CLARKE
OBE, MB, BS, DA, FFPM

With additional material by
FRANCIS COOKE

Edited by
JON PALETHORPE

POCKET REFERENCE BOOKS

A POCKET REFERENCE BOOK

Published by:
Pocket Reference Books Publishing Ltd.
Premier House
Hinton Road
Bournemouth
Dorset BH1 2EF

First Published 1996

Typesetting	Gary Tomlinson PrintRelate (Bournemouth, Dorset) (01202) 897659
Cover Design	Van Renselar Bonney Design Associates West Wickham, Kent BR4 9QH
Printing and Binding:	RPM Reprographics Units 2-3 Spur Road Quarry Lane, Chichester West Sussex PO19 2PR Tel. 01243 787077 Fax. 01243 780012 Modem 01243 536482 E-Mail: rpm@argonet.co.uk

ISBN 1 899437 20 7

Contents   Pages

ALL POCKET REFERENCE BOOKS INCLUDE A
FREE FULL PAGE ADVERTISEMENT ON THE
INSIDE FRONT COVER FOR A WELL-KNOWN CHARITY
SELECTED BY THE COMPILER

THE HISTORY OF THE CHARITY IS INCLUDED ON
THE INSIDE BACK COVER

The Publishers cannot be held responsible for any omissions or
information which is incorrect.
A very wide range of sources has been used by the compiler and the
editor, and the content of this Pocket Reference Book is dependent
upon the accuracy of those sources.

INTRODUCTION

Medical complaints have long been a source of fascination for the lay person, whether a stoic or a hypochondriac. This Pocket Reference Book is not meant to be a medical dictionary, which one would expect to cover a wider range of terminology. It is meant to be a source of specific medical diseases and conditions, some common, some less common, and some even obscure, as well as many of the signs and symptoms which go to make up those disease entities, such as headache, haematuria and dysphagia.

It is, however, a book which is intended to inform and not frighten!

The "fillers" provide potted biographies of some of the great historical names in medicine, from Hippocrates to Fleming and some medical complaints that may have altered the course of history. Dr. Clarke has also included anecdotes, both apocryphal and factual.

Whether or not Napoleon's piles did influence the Battle of Waterloo we shall now never know, but George III's bouts of insanity have been the subject of many learned articles in medical and historical journals. This Pocket Reference Book will be useful, not only to the layman, but also as an aide-memoire for those involved in paramedical specialities, as well as Pharmaceutical Representatives and Student Nurses. Even a copy in the pocket of the white coat of a Medical Student may help to keep him or her one step ahead of those medical or surgical tutors who take a sadistic delight in exposing that student's preference for being at a party the previous night rather than studying in the library! At least there were tutors like that around in the compiler's student days!

The information in this book is drawn from many sources, including the Readers' Digest Universal Dictionary, Black's Medical Dictionary, Longman's Pocket Medical Dictionary, the ABPI Expanded Syllabus, Encyclopaedia Britannica and other publications. One of the anecdotes are taken from the compiler's memory of stories published in World Medicine, a popular light medical journal of the 1960s and '70s.

A feature of the present day are the voluntary organisations which provide a source of information and support for sufferers of many chronic diseases. We have tried to provide a comprehensive list of these along with addresses and telephone numbers. If we have omitted any please let us know and we will try to include them in any future editions.

Dr. Clarke has produced an excellent Pocket Reference Book for the lay person, the medical student, the nurse, and for all those involved in caring for the sick, the elderly, the disabled – and even for the hypochondriac !

On examination the reader may find he or she is suffering from nothing at all !

L. GORDON

WHAT DO YOU KNOW ABOUT MEDICAL CONDITIONS?
TRY THESE TEASERS

Do you know how the Black Death was transmitted from China, where it began, to Europe?

Do you know who shook hands with an oak tree believing it was Frederick the Great of Prussia?

Do you know how Legionnaire's disease got its name?

Do you know that King George III's attacks of insanity are believed by medical historians to be due to a disorder of metabolism?

Do you know which English cricketer died from blood poisoning after a fall at a dance?

Do you know from which hereditary disease President Lincoln is believed to have suffered?

Do you know which London physician stopped a cholera epidemic by removing the handle of the Broad Street pump?

Do you know which Shakespearean hero 'was from his mother's womb untimely ripped'?

Do you know who discovered the circulation of the blood?

Do you know why Napoleon did not make his attack at Waterloo until midday?

You'll find the answers in the pages that follow

A

abortion – (miscarriage) the premature expulsion of a foetus from the womb; may be either spontaneous (most common 8-13 weeks) or induced.

abrasion – a rubbing of the surface of skin due to mechanical injury. Although slight, it can allow infection to enter.

abscess – a localised collection of pus. Acute ones develop rapidly and come up in a few days (e.g. boils). Chronic ones take weeks or months to develop (e.g tuberculosis).

acanthosis nigricans – dark pigmented verruca like skin change, often in the axilla and associated with cancer elsewhere in the body.

acapnia – a condition with reduced carbon dioxide in the blood.

achalasia – term for spasm, but more a failure to relax.

achalasia of the cardia – failure to relax muscles around the opening of oesophagus (gullet), where it enters the stomach.

achlorhydria – absence of hydrochloric acid in the stomach; associated with a number of diseases: e.g. pernicious anaemia, cancer of the stomach, gastritis.

achondroplasia – a shortening of arms and legs giving rise to dwarfism, an hereditary condition.

achylia gastrica – an absence of enzymes and hydrochloric acid in the stomach; food passes from the stomach to small intestine without undergoing digestion.

acidosis – diminution of the alkali reserve of the blood; occurs in some diseases of the kidney.

acne – (acne vulgaris) chronic skin condition affecting most adolescents; obstruction of ducts leading to sebaceous gland in skin, which become infected; activity of these glands are under the control of male sex hormones (secreted in testes in male and adrenal glands in female); predominantly affects face, back and chest.

aconite poisoning – poisoning by aconite (wolfsbane or monkshood).

acrocyanosis – condition in which there is persistent blueness of limbs, feet, nose and ears; usually occurs in women.

> "Every physician almost hath his favourite disease."
> From 'Tom Jones'
> (Henry Fielding 1707-1754)

acromegaly – overgrowth of bones of the limbs, feet, jaw and skull occurring after normal growth is complete; caused by increased secretion of growth hormone due to a tumour of anterior pituitary gland.

acroparaesthesia – disorder where there is numbness and tingling of fingers, particularly in women.

actinomycosis – acute or chronic suppurative disease affecting cattle, but can occur in man; caused by the fungus Actinomyces Israeli; the fungus can sometimes be found normally in the mouth, but following trauma to the mouth and jaw can give rise to abscesses; easily treatable with antibiotics.

adactyli – absence of digits.

Addison's disease – deficiency of hormones secreted by the adrenal cortex (adrenocorticoid hormone, aldosterone and androgens) due to its destruction. Originally, as described by Addison, due to tuberculosis; also due to auto-immune disease and secondary cancer.

adenitis – inflammation of a gland.

adenoiditis – inflammation of the adenoids.

adenoma – a benign tumour composed of glandular tissue.

adhesions – uniting of structures which should normally be separate and freely moving, resulting from acute or chronic inflammation.

adiposa dolorosa – (Dercan's disease) painful masses of fat developing under the skin, usually in women.

aerodontalgia – rare form of dental pain felt in restored non-vital teeth in those who fly.

aerophagy – name applied to the habit of air swallowing, especially in people suffering from dyspepsia.

afibrinogenaemia – condition in which blood fails to coagulate due to the absence of fibrin; can be congenital or acquired and gives rise to haemorrhage.

afterpains – pain occurring a few days after childbirth, similar to labour pains but not so severe; may be due to blood clots or pieces of placenta which the womb is trying to expel.

agammaglobulinaemia – childhood condition due to the absence of gamma globulin in the blood; makes the patient susceptible to infection.

agenesia – (agenesis) incomplete development of any part or organ of the body.

agnosia – loss of ability to recognise an object by any of the senses; occurs in various diseases of the brain.

agoraphobia – a sense of fear of being in large open spaces or going out in public. It can be a very distressing condition and advice can be obtained from the Phobics Society.

agranulocytosis – absence or greatly diminished numbers of white blood cells, either polymorpho-nuclear or granular types.

agraphia – loss of ability to express ideas by writing.

ague – a recurrent chill or fit of shivering, usually associated with malaria.

AIDS – acronym for acquired immunodeficiency syndrome; incurable disease caused by the human immunodeficiency virus, in which the ability to ward off infection is severely reduced. Transmitted by sexual activity (more commonly homosexual acts), infected syringes and blood products.

air sickness – form of motion sickness occurring in those travelling by air.

akinesia – loss or impairment of voluntary movement or mobility.

albinism – absence or a decrease in the amount of pigment, melanin, in the skin, hairs and eyes; inherited disease.

albuminuria – an excess amount of albumin in the urine, usually a sign of kidney or heart disease.

alcoholism (acute) – caused by taking a large quantity of alcohol over a short time; effects vary according to the person's constitution, e.g. unconsciousness, alcoholic mania, delirium tremens.

alcoholism (chronic) – caused by taking too much alcohol over a long period; important to differentiate between chronic alcoholism and heavy drinkers; the latter can stop, a chronic alcoholic can't, without help; effects include brain damage, liver damage and delirium tremens.

aldosteronism – a form of treatable high blood pressure with weakness, headaches and other symptoms, due to an excessive production of aldosterone, a salt regulating enzyme produced by the adrenal cortex.

Aleppo evil – see oriental sore.

alexia – another name for dyslexia or word blindness.

algid – the state in malaria or cholera where extreme coldness of the body occurs.

alkalosis – a decrease in the concentration of hydrogen ions in the blood making it more alkaline; can occur if large amounts of alkaline compounds are taken for the treatment of a stomach ulcer.

alkaptonuria – a rare hereditary disorder, where the body is incapable of producing the enzymes which enable it to make proper use of some of the amino acids in protein foods; the by-products of incomplete metabolism cause the urine to turn dark on standing; in later life it causes discolouration of cartilage and may lead to severe arthritis.

allantiasis – sausage poisoning.

allergy – abnormal reaction to certain substances, which would cause no symptoms in most people, e.g. certain foods, pollen, insect bites; symptoms include asthma, dyspepsia, nettle rash, hay fever, eczema and headaches; substances producing it are known as allergens, which produce antibodies causing the release of the histamine bradykinin.

allocheiria – a disorder of sensation, where the sensations are referred to the wrong part of the body.

alopecia – another name for baldness.

alopecia areata – a disorder where the hair comes out in patches.

alveolitis – inflammation of the alveoli (air sacs) of the lungs caused by an allergic reaction; when caused by infection it is called pneumonia.

Alzheimer's disease – degenerative disorder of the cerebral cortex producing dementia in middle or late life; the first manifestation is failing memory, particularly for recent events.

> **ALOIS ALZHEIMER** was a German neuropathologist who, in 1906, described two abnormalities of the brain in a patient of 55 who died of severe dementia.
>
> Firstly he observed plaques on nervous tissue, which had previously been described in the brains of elderly people, and secondly he noted a tangle of fibrous tissue within nerve cells which showed up when stained with silver.
>
> This latter discovery had not been described before and it was this that defined a new disease entity.
>
> Because of the relatively young age of this patient Alzheimer's disease was long regarded as a form of presenile dementia, but as it is now recognised that the same pathological atrophy is also present in patients of an advanced age, most authorities no longer restrict the term to presenile cases.

amaurosis – blindness in which there is no obvious lesion in the eye; disease of the optic nerve, retina, brain or hysteria. (Burns' amaurosis is described as a dimness of vision due to sexual excess!).

amaurosis fugax – sudden transitory blindness or impaired vision, possibly due to circulatory failure; can occur in migraine.

ambivalence – psychological state where the person loves and hates a person or object at the same time.

ambylopia – defective vision with no organic lesion in the eye; may be due to defective development, hysteria, excess alcohol or other toxins; the commonest form is associated with squints.

amelia – absence of limbs, usually congenital.

amenorrhoea – absence of menstrual flow during the time of life at which this should occur; a sign in many medical conditions, but the commonest cause is pregnancy.

amentia – mental deficiency from a failure of the mind to develop normally.

ametropia – an error of refraction through the lens of an eye.

amnesia – loss of memory.

amoebiasis – infestation by the protozoa Entamoeba histolytica giving rise to amoebic dysentery; complications include perforation of the intestine, haemorrhaging into the gut, abscesses in the liver, brain, bones and testes.

amputee – someone who has a limb or a part of a limb removed.

amyloidosis – abnormal masses of protein infiltrating various organs; either primary or secondary to chronic disease, e.g. tuberculosis.

amyotonia – lack of muscle tone.

amyotrophic lateral sclerosis – a disease of the spinal cord producing progressive paralysis and a wasting of muscles on either side of the body.

> **anaemia** – a condition caused by an inadequate number of red blood corpuscles or amount of haemoglobin in the blood; a number of varieties exist (described under their individual titles).

anaphylaxis – excessive sensitivity by certain people to an injection of foreign material or substance; extreme form of allergy can give rise to shortness of breath, acute urticaria, angioneurotic oedema, low blood pressure and, in extreme cases, death.

ancylostomiasis – parasitic infestation by the hookworm.

anencephaly – rare condition where a child is born with a defect in the skull and absence of brain.

aneuploidy – condition where there is an abnormal number of chromosomes, e.g. mongolism, Turner's syndrome.

aneurysm – a blood filled sac formed by dilation of artery walls making it susceptible to rupture and haemorrhage; can occur in different arteries, e.g. the aorta, the small arteries of the brain. A communication between an artery and vein is known as an arterio-venous aneurysm.

angiitis – inflammation of the blood or lymph vessel.

angina – literally means 'choking', swelling of throat and other forms of difficulty in breathing; used more as a general term referring to angina pectoris.

angina pectoris – a crushing or gripping pain in the chest, usually related to exertion or excitement; caused by insufficient blood passing through the coronary arteries, giving rise to oxygen lack in the heart muscle.

angioma – tumour composed of blood vessels.

angioneurotic oedema – acute local swelling under the skin often as a result of food allergy, similar to nettle rash; serious if it occurs around the tongue or larynx, where it could give rise to suffocation.

anhidrosis – abnormal deficiency in the secretion of sweat.

ankylosing spondylitis – inflammatory condition, involving vertebrae, of the spine, most common in males aged 20-40; vertebrae become 'bamboo' shaped, causing fixation of spine and leading to boney fusion.

ankylosis – a condition of joints, where movements are restricted by fibrous bands, malformation or fusion. It may be a deliberate surgical procedure to produce immobilisation.

anorexia – loss of appetite.

anorexia nervosa – nervous disorder, predominantly in girls, manifested by a deep aversion to food; often starts when there is a mistaken belief that the person is overweight, leading to dieting to excess; the condition leads to extreme emaciation.

anosmia – loss of the sense of smell.

anoxaemia – reduction of oxygen content in the blood.

anteflexion – abnormal forward curvature of an organ.

anthracosis – changes that have taken place in the lungs and bronchi; occurs in coalminers and others who inhale coal dust.

> **anthrax** – serious disease occurring principally in sheep and cattle and also in those who tend them or handle the bones, skin and fleeces; sometimes known as 'wool sorter's disease'; caused by a bacillus (B. anthracis), giving rise to infected ulcers particularly on the face or arm.

anuria – condition where no urine is passed, due to suppression of urine secretion.

anxiety state – another name for anxiety neurosis.

aortitis – degenerative condition of the aorta, usually a complication of syphilis.

aphakia – absence of the lens of the eye.

aphasia – loss of the power of speech due to injury or disease of that part of the brain.

> "Time is the great physician."
> Benjamin Disraeli (1804-1881)

aphonia – loss of voice usually due to a disorder of the throat.

aplastic anaemia – serious form of anaemia due to the failure of the bone marrow to form new blood cells; can be caused by chemicals (including some drugs) which poison the cell producing mechanisms of the bone marrow.

apnoea – temporary stoppage of breathing due to a lack of stimulation of the breathing centre in the brain.

apodia – absence of a foot.

apoplexy – a stroke.

appendicitis – inflammation of the appendix.

apraxia – loss of the power to carry out regulated movements.

arachnodactyly – also known as Marfan's syndrome; a rare hereditary disease characterised by an extreme length of fingers and toes, disproportionally long legs, flabby tissues, funnel chest or pigeon breast, flat feet, displacement of the lens of the eye; fundamental defect believed to be in the connective tissue. Evidence suggests that Abraham Lincoln was a sufferer.

arcus senilis – a white ring around the outer edge of the cornea of the eye particularly in the aged.

> **Argyll Robertson pupil** – a condition of the eye where the pupil reacts to accommodation but not to light; a feature of syphilis of the central nervous system.

argyria – the effects of taking silver substances in excess over time.

arrhythmia – variation from the normal rhythm of the heartbeat.

arsenic poisoning – poisoning by compounds of arsenic.

arteriosclerosis – a thickening and hardening of the walls of the arteries, particularly the medium sized ones, leading to loss of elasticity; a natural change in old age.

arterio-venous aneurysm – abnormal communication between an artery and a vein; can be the result of a gunshot wound.

arteritis – inflammatory condition of an artery.

arthritis – inflammation of the joints.

arthropathy – term applied to any form of joint disease.

asbestosis – slowly progressive inflammation of the lungs resulting from the inhalation of asbestos fibres; it occurs in miners and workers in trades exposed to materials containing asbestos fibres; can lead to a form of cancer of the lung.

ascariasis – infestation with round worms.

ascites – accumulation of fluid in the abdominal cavity, also known as 'dropsy'.

aspergillosis – a disease due to the invasion of the lungs by the fungus Aspergillus fumigatus; the air-borne spores are inhaled and the fungus grows in damaged parts of the lung, e.g. tuberculous cavities, abscesses or dilated bronchioles as in bronchiectasis.

asphyxia – means literally absence of pulse, but it refers to a whole series of symptoms following the stoppage of breathing and the action of the heart following; death occurs due to insufficient oxygen taken up by the blood.

asphyxia neonatorum – a condition where there is imperfect breathing in the newborn.

asteriognosis – loss of the capacity to recognise the nature of an object by feeling it. It indicates the presence of a lesion, e.g. a tumour, in the brain.

asthenia – a lack of strength.

asthenopia – a weakness in the eyes caused by long-sightedness, inflammation or weakness of the eye muscles.

asthma – a disorder of respiration where there are paroxysms of difficult, wheezy breathing; usually an allergic reaction causing spasmodic contraction of the smaller bronchial tubes and can be made worse by lung damage or chronic or repeated infection.

astigmatism – an error of refraction in the cornea or lens of the eye; objects appear distorted.

asynergia – a sign of some diseases of the nervous system where there is an absence of harmonious and coordinated movements between muscles which have opposite actions.

ataxia – a loss of coordination ; although the power to make movement is present, these are undisciplined; present in sensory defects of the nervous system or in diseases affecting the cerebellum.

atelectasis – collapse of all or part of a lung; may be due to an obstruction of part of the bronchial tree, e.g. by inhalation of a foreign body like a peanut.

atheroma – degenerative condition of the inner coat of an artery, where plaques of yellowish material are deposited, made up of cholesterol and other fatty substances; causes the lumen of the artery to become smaller.

athetosis – usually occurs in children due to brain disease or damage; consists of slow involuntary writhing movements of the fingers, toes or other parts.

athlete's foot – a skin eruption of the foot most commonly between the toes; usually due to a fungus infection (ringworm).

atony – a lack of tone in muscles and other organs.

atopy – a form of allergy which is inherited, including asthma, hay fever and eczema.

> "Honour a physician with the honour due unto him for the uses which ye may of him; for the Lord hath created him!"
>
> From Eccliasticus.

atresia – absence of a natural opening to an organ.

atrophy – a state of wasting away or shrinking in size of a tissue, organ or a part.

aura – a peculiar feeling or premonition in persons before the occurrence of an epileptic fit.

autism – a disharmony in development in which children are unable to mature socially despite good motor skills.

auto-immunity – the development of antibodies to one's own tissue; occurs in diseases like rheumatoid arthritis.

auto-intoxication – self poisoning by substances formed in the body.

automatism – the performance of acts without being conscious of them e.g. after an epileptic fit before regaining consciousness, sleeping; the person has no memory of having performed the act.

auto-suggestion – a mental condition which can occur after an accident or injury; slight or temporary injury is exaggerated, the person thinking that there is serious disability like blindness.

avitaminosis – a condition where there is a deprivation of vitamins.

azoospermia – absence of active spermatazoa in the semen.

azotaemia – the presence of urea and other nitrogenous compounds in excess amounts in the blood; it occurs in severe kidney disease.

backache – symptom of many diseases ranging from local injury to the back and local disease to referred pain from diseases in deep seated organs.

bacteraemia – condition of which bacteria are present in the blood; a transient form can occur following extraction of a tooth.

bacteruria – presence of bacteria in the urine; usually a sign of infection in the kidneys, bladder or urethra.

bagassosis – industrial lung disease in those who work with bagasse, the name given to the broken sugar cane after sugar has been extracted. Bagasse contains silica, therefore the disease is a form of silicosis.

balanitis – inflammation of the part of the penis covered by the prepuce or foreskin.

balantidiasis – a form of dysentery caused by the protozoa Balantidium coli (a common parasite in the pig).

balbuties – a term for stammering.

baldness – loss of hair (see alopecia).

Banti's disease – a type of anaemia associated with enlargement of the spleen (splenic anaemia).

baragnosis – a condition associated with some diseases of the brain, where the individual is unable to appreciate that an object placed in the hand has weight.

barber's itch – the hair follicles, particularly around the chin, become infected, usually by a staphylococcus or ringworm; believed to come from infected barbers' implements; otherwise known as sycosis barbi.

> **Basedow's disease** – another name for Graves' disease or exophthalmic goitre (thyrotoxicosis); can be caused by auto-immunity.

basophilia – an increase in the number of basophils (a type of white blood corpuscle) in the blood.

bat ears – term applied to prominent ears.

bather's itch – rash on the skin appearing on those who bathe in water infected with the larvae of the schistosome trematode worm; it is carried by snails particularly in the U.S, Canada, Central and South America, Australia, Malaysia and Japan.

beat elbow – term used by miners who suffer from inflamed elbows (also beat knee and hand); caused by the constant use of a tool or pressure due to resting on the joints at work.

Bechet's syndrome – oral and genital ulceration, inflammation of the iris and ciliary body of the eye (iridocyclitis), painful joints, thrombophlebitis and sometimes involvement of the central nervous system.

bed sores – sores or ulcers occurring in pressure areas of the body, particularly in the lower part of the back, usually in those confined to bed and weakened by disease; also known as decubitus ulcers.

bee sting – a sting by a bee; can produce a severe allergic reaction in susceptible individuals.

Bell's palsy – paralysis of the muscles of the face on one or both sides due to damage or inflammation of the facial nerve (VIIth cranial nerve); if due to inflammation the paralysis is usually temporary; if due to damage it may be permanent.

> **bends** – affects those who work in compressed air, e.g. underwater divers; caused by the accumulation of bubbles of nitrogen in different parts of the body when decompression takes place too quickly (also known as caisson disease).

Bennett's fracture – longitudinal fracture of the first metacarpal bone, also affecting the carpo-metacarpal joint.

beriberi – a disease caused by a deficiency in vitamin B1 (thiamine) due to eating highly polished rice; dry beriberi affects the nerves of the extremities and wet beriberi causes dropsy and heart failure; most common in Japan, Malaysia, Fiji, India and West Africa.

beryllosis – lung disease caused by the inhalation of beryllium oxide.

bilharziasis – another form of schistosomiasis.

bird fancier's lung – allergic inflammation of the alveoli of the lung in those sensitive to pigeon or other bird's droppings, feathers and eggs.

birth mark – a mark, stain or mole present from birth.

black death – old name for bubonic plague.

black fat tobacco disease – a form of pneumonia caused by smoking black fat tobacco (tobacco flavoured with canopus oil); only reported in Guyana.

blackwater fever – acute illness with haemoglobin present in the urine, jaundice, fever, anaemia and vomiting; associated with malignant tertian malaria.

blenhorrhoea – the excessive discharge of slimy material from a surface e.g. eye, nose, bowel; similar to catarrh but not obviously infected.

blepharitis – inflammation of the eyelid.

blepharospasm – repeated twitching or even closure of the eyelid due to spasm of muscle surrounding the eye.

blighted ovum – after fertilisation normal development of embryo occurs for short time and then dies; membranes live longer – probably caused by an abnormal foetus in the womb.

blindness – lack of vision where the acuity is less than 6/60 in the better eye, but if the acuity is better, where the field of vision is markedly contracted in the greater part of its extent. Defined in 1948 National Assistance Act as 'so blind as to be unable to perform any work for which eyesight is essential'.

blisters – lesions on the surface of the skin filled with straw coloured fluid.

blood poisoning – known as septicaemia or pyaemia, where micro-organisms circulate in the blood; abscesses can be formed in parts of the body; a serious condition often fatal before the advent of antibiotics.

> W.W. 'Dodge' Whysall, the Nottinghamshire and England cricketer, slipped and grazed his elbow at a dance in Mansfield in the early winter of 1930. Blood poisoning (septicaemia) set in and he died on November 11th. Today he would have been treated by antibiotics and would have lived to play another season.

boil – type of abscess occurring on the skin, usually starting in the root of hair follicles; usually due to infection caused by Staphylococcus aureus; also known as a furuncle; when a number come together it is known as a carbuncle.

borborygmus – flatulence, causing noises in the bowel.

Bornholm disease – epidemic condition associated with acute pain in the muscles around the lower margin of the ribs; more common in young males and in warm weather; lasts seven to ten days and is named after an island in the Baltic where epidemics have been reported. Sometimes known as 'devil's grip'.

> **botulism** – rare but extremely severe form of food poisoning caused by a spore bearing organism, Clostridium botulinum; the condition starts by producing acute abdominal pain and vomiting progressing on to nervous system symptoms; it has a high mortality rate of over 50%; the organism grows in badly preserved or canned food.

Bowen's disease – a genetic form of carcinoma found in the skin; there is abnormal keratin in the hair follicles and an isolated scaling plaque on the skin.

bow legs – a bowing of the legs possibly due to an abnormal posture of the limbs in the womb; in older children it can be due to bone disease e.g. rickets.

brachycephalic – a shortness of the head, a feature of some alpine races.

brachydactyly – a condition in which fingers or toes are abnormally short.

bradycardia – slow heart beat.

bradykinesis – a condition in which the movements of the body and limbs are abnormally slow.

breakbone fever – a name for dengue.

breathlessness – any condition where the blood is impure and short of oxygen, making it necessary to produce excessive voluntary effort to gain more air.

Bright's disease – a progressive disease of the kidneys affecting the glomerulus (a fine tuft of small blood vessels making up part of the filtering mechanism); usually proceeds to renal failure. Patients suffer from oedema, albumen in the urine and high blood pressure; otherwise known as glomerulonephritis.

brittle bone disease – inherited abnormality where extreme fragility of the skeleton results in recurrent fractures; other deformities of the bones occur, also blue sclera (normally white part of the eye), transparent teeth, and deafness, otherwise known as osteitis imperfecta.

bromhidrosis – excretion of evil smelling perspiration.

bromism – due to the ingestion of too much bromide giving rise to acne of the face, mental dullness, sleepiness, weakness, unsteady gait and bad breath.

bronchiectasis – condition whereby the bronchi become dilated usually as a result of recurrent infection of the bronchial tree. The bronchi become obstructed by the infection. Other causes include tuberculosis, cancer or inhalation of a foreign body. It becomes difficult to get rid of the secretions. Affects the bronchi and bronchioles and can be an after-effect of infection due to measles and whooping cough.

bronchitis – inflammation of the bronchi; can be acute or chronic; chronic bronchitis occurs following repeated attacks of the acute variety and usually occurs in elderly people.

brow ague – frontal neuralgia, tic dolorosa or neuralgia; associated with migraine.

brucellosis – an infectious disease transferred from animals to man (Malta or undulant fever); mostly caused by contact with cattle or by consuming raw dairy products; infection by the organism Brucella melitenis (goats' milk) and Brucella abortus (cows' milk); the fever is undulating sometimes with an enlarged spleen or liver. Causes contagious abortion in cattle; most common in Malta and other Mediterranean islands.

bruise – contusion affecting skin and the tissue underneath; the colour is due to the outpouring of blood from ruptured vessels into a confined space.

> "They that be whole need not a physician, but they that are sick."
>
> St Matthew

bruxism – habit of grinding the teeth usually while asleep and being unaware of it.

bubo – swelling of lymphatic glands in the groin due to plague or venereal disease.

bubonic plague – infectious epidemic disease occurring in man and lower animals.

The organism causing it is Yersinia (formally known as Pasteurella) pestis which is transferred to man by the bite of the flea of the black rat (Rattus rattus); gives rise to fever and swollen glands of the groin; if it goes on to affect the lungs (pneumonic) or the bloodstream (septicaemic) it can prove rapidly fatal.

Endemic in parts of China, India and East Africa – last cases in the U.K. in Suffolk; responsible for the Black Death.

THE BLACK DEATH

The Black Death which swept across Europe in the 14th century consisted of both the bubonic and pneumonic plague.

It originated in China and was transmitted to Europe in 1347 during the siege of a Genoese trading post in the Crimea, when the besieging army catapulted plague infected corpses into the town.

Over 25 million of the population of Europe are believed to have died from the plague.

Not even the great and good were spared and victims included Eleanor of Aragon, King Alfonso XI of Castile and Joan, daughter of Edward III, who died on the way to her wedding to Alfonso's son.

Two successive Archbishops of Canterbury, during Edward's reign, also succumbed.

The great plague of London in 1665 accounted for 70,000 deaths out of the population of 460,000.

Buerger's disease – named after the American surgeon who first described the condition (thromboangitis obliterans); caused by narrowing of the arteries leading to the limbs, particularly the legs; the use of tobacco is an important factor; more common in middle European Jews; produces increasing pain in the legs on walking, which ceases on stopping ('intermittent claudication' from the Latin claudio – I limp); can lead to ulceration of legs, hands and feet and gangrene.

bulimia – insatiable appetite of psychological origin.

bulimia nervosa – an overpowering urge to eat large amounts of food followed by self induced vomiting or the abuse of laxatives; there is a morbid fear of obesity as in anorexia nervosa; most common in women in their twenties.

bulla – another word for blister.

bunions – also known as hallux valgus; the big joint of the big toe becomes enlarged and thickened and bends inwards towards the little toe; can become inflamed due to the joint rubbing on the shoe; surgical correction may be necessary.

Burkitt's lymphoma – a form of malignant tumour usually affecting the jaw and facial bones; most often found in children of Central Africa; disease responds well to therapy and is thought to be caused by the Epstein-Barr virus.

bursitis – inflammation of a bursa, which is a sac between joints or moving surfaces in the body.

byssinosis – an occupational disease of textile workers caused by inhaling dust during the processing stages in cotton, flax and hemp mills; thought to be due to a chemical substance in textile dusts which constricts the bronchi and causes asthma type symptoms.

cachexia – weakness, emaciation and general ill-health resulting from a serious disease such as cancer.

cadaveric rigidity – another name for rigor mortis.

cadmium poisoning – a hazard in certain industrial processes e.g. the manufacture of cadmium plating. Cadmium is present in sewage sludge, which is used as a fertiliser, therefore vegetables may become contaminated; symptoms include stomach pains, diarrhoea and vomiting.

caesarian section – delivery of a child by opening the abdomen and womb from the front. It was believed that caesarian section was so called because Julius Caesar was born thus; more likely named because under caesarean law it was forbidden to bury a pregnant woman until her baby had been removed. In Shakespeare, Macbeth was told 'none of woman born shall harm Macbeth'. Macduff said; 'Macduff was from his mother's womb untimely ripped'. Perhaps Macduff was born by caesarian section?

caisson disease – see bends.

café au lait spots – multiple pigmented areas on the skin, the colour of café au lait; present in neurofibromatosis.

calcicosis – disease of the lung caused by the inhalation of marble dust, in marble cutters.

calculus – stone or concretion which may be found in the bladder, kidney or gallbladder.

callosities – thickening of the outer layers of the skin or epidermis.

cancer – or carcinoma; general names for forms of malignant tumours, which invade and destroy tissues; cancer named after the Latin for crab – a sort of 'creeping ulcer'.

cancrum oris – gangrenous ulcer around the mouth affecting weakly children after a severe disease like measles; bacteria grow in the tissues affected.

candida – otherwise known as candidiasis or moniliasis; infection due to the fungus, Candida albicans; occurs in the mouth and vagina (thrush), where it is the most common fungus infection; presents as white patches and discharge; also occurs in the skin folds and on the vulva; may occur after a prolonged course of antibiotics or when the body's immune system is compromised.

canities – a whitening or greying of the hair.

canker – small ulcer around the mouth or lips due to local irritation or in conditions causing dyspepsia and general ill-health.

caput medusae – abnormal dilated veins around the umbilicus in cirrhosis of the liver.

caput succedaneum – temporary swelling sometimes found on the head of a new born infant.

carbolic acid poisoning – may be accidental or suicidal; causes burning about the mouth and throat followed by numbness; white ulcers present on the mucus membranes of the mouth where the acid has burned; if untreated, unconsciousness, stupor and death follow within a few hours.

carbon monoxide poisoning – may be accidental or suicidal; due to faulty or deliberate turning on of a gas fire or from the exhaust of a car; carbon monoxide replaces oxygen in the blood forming carboxyhaemoglobin.

> **carbuncle** – deep seated infection of the skin, like several boils joined together; pus is discharged from a number of points on the tight reddened skin; the infection usually due to a staphylococcus.

cardiac asthma – paroxysms of difficult breathing, often occurring at night; characteristic of congestive cardiac failure, where fluid congregates in the lungs; very different from bronchial asthma.

cardiospasm – spasmodic contraction of muscle surrounding the opening of the oesophagus into the stomach.

caries – dental decay where the calcified structure of the tooth is removed by disease; may be due to bacterial action by the organism Streptococcus mutans.

carneous mole – an ovum which has died in the early months of pregnancy.

carpal tunnel syndrome – attacks of pain and tingling in the first three or four fingers in one or both hands (worse at night); caused by pressure on the median nerve as it passes under the ligament that lies across the wrist.

car sickness – motion sickness in those travelling by car.

caruncle – a small non-malignant fleshy growth which can be normal or abnormal; one type occurs at the urinary outlet of women (urethral caruncle), causing pain and bleeding.

caseation – a process which takes place in tissues in chronic inflammatory diseases, particularly tuberculosis, where the central part of an area changes into pus forming an abscess; this then forms a cheese-like mass, which eventually heals by becoming calcified.

castration – operation for removal of testicles or ovaries.

catalepsy – a nervous condition with sudden suspension of volition accompanied by a peculiar rigidity of the whole part of the body or of certain muscles; can occur in epilepsy, hysteria, encephalitis or schizophrenia; a statue like appearance of the body.

catamenia – another term for menstruation.

cataplexy – condition in which patient has a sudden attack of muscular weakness affecting the whole body (a temporary paralysis).

> **cataract** – an opacity of the lens of the eye which may be age related, due to trauma or metabolic diseases such as diabetes; untreated it gets increasingly severe leading to blindness; cataracts can be congenital (e.g. due to rubella) or inherited. Treated by surgery.

catarrh – a state of irritation of the mucous membranes, particularly those of the air passages; there is a copious secretion of mucus which becomes purulent following infection of the upper respiratory tract. Taste and smell become impaired and if the eustachian tubes become blocked it can cause infection of the middle ear.

catatonia – a mental condition in which the patient remains rigidly in the same position like a statue, a state in schizophrenia. Related to catalepsy.

catatonia minor – a group of symptoms occurring in schizophrenia where the patient displays peculiar mannerisms such as repeating the same words or actions.

cat scratch fever – probably a virus infection associated with enlargement of the glands; in spite of its name a history of a cat scratch is only present in about half of the cases; can occur following the puncture of the skin by a splinter or thorn; the glandular swelling is usually short term, but can proceed to abscess formation.

cauliflower ear – term applied to the distortion of the external ear by repeated injury, usually in sport; it starts as a haematoma in the auricle.

cellulitis – wide spread septic inflammation of the soft loose connective tissue under the skin.

cement burns – burns caused by prolonged contact of the skin with builders cement (due to quicklime in the cement mixture).

cerebral palsy – a group of diseases with various degrees of paralysis occurring in infancy or early childhood; paralysis may be flaccid but in 80% it is spastic (hence the term 'spastics'); may be genetic due to a congenital defect of the brain or to trauma at childbirth.

cerebrospinal fever – another name for cerebrospinal meningitis.

cerebro vascular accident – another name for a stroke.

cervicitis – inflammation of the neck of the womb.

Chadwick's sign – a blue discolouration around the entrance to the vagina and on the neck of the uterus; an early sign of pregnancy.

chafing of the skin – occurs in infants at the natural folds in the groin, armpits or on the elbow where two moist surfaces rub together; also occurs in stout elderly people.

Chagas' disease – American trypanosomiasis; caused by the protozoan organism Trypanosoma cruri transmitted by biting bugs in Central and South America; it can be acute or chronic; the acute form is common in children affecting the heart while the chronic form usually occurs in adolescents and young adults; the outcome depends on the extent of heart damage. It can give rise to permanent chronic illness; it is believed to have affected Charles Darwin on his voyage on the 'Beagle' turning him into a chronic invalid and being ultimately responsible for his death.

chalazion – a cyst of the meibomiam gland of the eyelid which can be single or multiple; they may become chronically inflamed.

chancre – a primary lesion of syphilis.

chancroid – soft non-syphilitic venereal sore due to the bacterium Haemophilus ducreyi.

chapped hands – occur in cold weather when the activity of the sweat and sebaceous glands becomes reduced providing less natural protection and the skin becomes cracked and inelastic. A similar state can occur on the lips and nipples.

Charcot's joints – painless swelling and disorganisation of the joints as a result of damage to the pain fibres. Occurs in tabes dorsalis, a condition of the nervous system caused by tertiary syphilis, and diabetic neuritis.

JEAN MARTIN CHARCOT (1825-1893) was one of France's greatest medical teachers and clinicians as well as being one of the founders of modern neurology. His neurological clinic, opened in 1882, attracted students from all around the world, one of his students being Sigmund Freud. He was the first to describe the disintegration of ligaments and joint surfaces caused by locomotor ataxia, a manifestation of tertiary syphilis, and referred to as Charcot's joint. Charcot also discovered miliary aneurysms (the dilation of small arteries supplying the brain) and their importance in haemorrhage (see sub-arachnoid haemorrhage). Charcot's joint was not, as bawdy medical students might have believed, a night club, but a complication of syphilis!

cheilosis – eczematous condition of the lips, especially at the angle of the mouth, due to deficiency of vitamin B$_2$ (riboflavin).

cheiropompholyx – disease of the skin in which small blisters, filled with clear fluid, sometimes appear on the hands.

chicken pox – an acute, highly infectious fever characterised by the appearance of a rash consisting of successive crops of vesicles, occurring mainly in children.

chilblain – an acute or chronic form of cold 'injury'; less severe than frostbite, in which there is inflammation of the skin, itching, swelling and sometimes blisters.

child-crowing – another name for spasm of the larynx in children.

chincough – another name for whooping cough.

chloasma – an increase in melanin pigment in the skin as a result of hormonal stimulation.

chloroma – (green cancer) a disease in which green growths appear under the skin with changes, similar to leukaemia, occurring in the blood.

> **chlorosis** – a form of iron deficiency anaemia chiefly affecting young girls around puberty, characterised by yellowish or greenish grey complexion. Not often seen now but common before First World War – associated with fainting ('swooning'!)

choking – the process associated with an obstruction to breathing in the larynx. It can be caused by a swelling around the glottis (the entrance to the larynx), a nervous disorder interfering with the muscles surrounding it or, more commonly, due to the inhalation of a foreign body e.g. food 'going down the wrong way'.

cholangitis – inflammation of the bile ducts.

cholecystitis – inflammation of the gallbladder.

cholelithiasis – the presence of gall stones.

> **cholera** – epidemic disease caused by the ingestion of the organism Vibrio cholerae, which is transmitted in the bowel discharges of carriers to food and water. It produces profuse watery diarrhoea (rice water stools), cramps, vomiting, prostration and suppression of urine. In severe cases death is caused by extreme dehydration. Outbreaks occur mainly in India, Pakistan, Bangladesh and South East Asia. Vaccination gives some immunity for a short time. The water-borne nature of the disease was discovered by the London physician John Snow, in 1854, when he ordered the closure of the Broad Street pump, which ended an epidemic in the area of London served by that pump.

JOHN SNOW (1813 – 1858), a York born London physician, who was a pioneer of the science of anaesthesia, spent much of his time in the mid-nineteenth century researching the way cholera was spread.

During one epidemic he noted that most of those succumbing to the disease drew their water supply from the pump in Broad Street in the City of London. He ordered that the handle of the pump be removed. The spread of this disease in this epidemic ceased.

There was, however, one mystery. An elderly lady who lived in Hampstead, an area not supplied from the Broad Street pump, also died from cholera in the epidemic.

On investigation, Snow discovered that the old lady had lived near Broad Street and she preferred the flavour of the water from that pump to that which was available in Hampstead. Consequently she sent her maid every day down to Broad Street to draw a bucket of her favourite water.

This research convinced Snow that cholera was a water-borne disease.

chondroma – a tumour composed mainly of cartilage.

chorea – a disease of the nervous system marked by involuntary, irregular rapid, jerky movements of the muscles of the face, legs and arms. The commonest form, Sydenhams' chorea or St. Vitus dance is a disease of childhood, often associated with rheumatic fever. The jerky movements usually subside within a few weeks.

choriocarcinoma – cancer affecting the chorion which is the external of the two foetal membranes.

choroiditis – inflammation of the middle coat of the eye.

Christmas disease – an hereditary disorder of blood coagulation due to a shortage of one of the clotting factors (factor IX); similar to haemophilia but the deficiency is of a different blood clotting factor. Named after the surname of the first recorded patient.

cicatrix – another name for a scar.

circumcision – surgical removal of foreskin or prepuce.

cirrhosis of the liver – chronic progressive inflammation of the liver with increasing amounts of non–functioning fibrous tissue replacing the normal tissue. The organ can become enlarged or shrivelled and eventually ceases to function. Complications include oedema, digestive complaints, weight loss, jaundice and bleeding of the veins of the oesophagus. It can be a complication of hepatitis and chronic alcoholism.

chyluria – passage of chyle (milky fluid absorbed from the lymph vessels of the intestine) in the urine; a manifestation of filariasis, an infestation by the parasite Filaria bancrofti, which obstructs the lymphatics.

claustrophobia – fear of being in a confined space.

claw foot – (pes cavus), familial condition characterised by an abnormally high arch of foot with shortening of the toes and inversion or turning inwards of the foot and heel, giving rise to pain and a stiff gait.

claw hand – a bending and wasting of the hand and fingers (especially ring and little finger) usually due to paralysis of the ulnar nerve. It can also be caused by contact pressure of a tool against the hand leading to contraction of the fibrous tissue.

cleft palate – a congenital malformation of the lip, palate or both when they fail to fuse properly in the midline during foetal development. They normally fuse about the eighth week of pregnancy. Modern plastic surgery and early diagnosis gives the condition a much better outlook; incidence about 1 in 700.

clicking finger – occurs in middle age when the ring or middle finger cannot be straightened spontaneously on awakening; can only straighten with a special effort and a painful click; caused by a swelling developing in one of the tendons.

clonic – a word applied to short spasmodic movements.

clubbing the fingers – thickening and broadening of the finger tips, with overhanging nails, resulting from a local shortage of oxygenated blood; usually associated with certain diseases of the heart and lungs e.g. emphysema, bronchiectasis, cancer of the lung and congenital conditions.

> **club foot** – otherwise called talipes. A condition whereby the foot is permanently twisted at the ankle joint with the sole no longer resting on the ground when standing; it is believed to be due to a fixed position of the foetus in the womb maintained for a long period of foetal life. If the sufferer walks on the outer edge of the foot it is called talipes varus, if on the inner edge, talipes valgus. The Emperor Claudius, so called from the Latin word to limp (see Buerger's disease) was born with a clubfoot.

cluster headaches – sometimes called migrainous neuralgia, but a different condition from migraine. The headaches appear in periods of 6–12 weeks at certain times of the year and usually affect one side and often occur around the eye.

coal miner's lung – see anthracosis.

coarctation of the aorta – a congenital constriction of the aorta, the large blood vessel carrying blood away from the heart.

coccydynia – severe pain in the coccyx, which is at the lower end of the spine.

coeliac disease – a wasting disease of childhood due to the inability to absorb fat through the small intestine wall, hence an excess of fat is found in the stools; it is due to the intolerance of gluten a constituent of wheat flour, which causes damage to the lining of the small intestine.

cold sores – see herpes simplex.

colitis – inflammation of the colon.

collagen disease – a term used to describe a group of diseases, including acute rheumatism and rheumatoid arthritis, in which changes occur in the collagen of the tissues.

collapse – a condition of extreme weakness of all body powers especially the nervous system; it is the terminal state of many severe diseases. It can occur in severe surgical shock.

Colles' fracture – a fracture of the lower end of the radius close to the wrist, caused by a fall on the wrist; the lower fragment of the bone is displaced backwards.

colostomy – a surgically created opening of the colon through the wall of the abdomen to form an artificial anus.

colour blindness – a condition which can occur in the presence of normal visual acuity; it can be either hereditary or acquired and is more common in men (7% of the population) than women (0.5%). In the hereditary form the women carry the affected gene, which is passed to their offspring. Red/green colour blindness is most common. The acquired form is the result of a disease of the cones or their connections in the retina.

colpitis – inflammation of the vagina.

coma – a state of profound or deep unconsciousness, where the sufferer cannot be roused; there is no reflex movement when the skin is pinched. Caused by many conditions e.g. head injury, strokes, poisoning, tumours, diabetes, severe liver and kidney disease, diabetes and epilepsy, to mention a few.

commotio cerebri – concussion of the brain.

compositor's disease – a form of lead poisoning affecting those who handle metal type.

concussion – may result from a fall or violent blow in which the brain receives a jarring or shaking; the injured person may or may not be knocked out but may be dizzy, sleepy, nauseated and have a cold skin and pallor.

condyloma – a warty growth on the skin around the anus or external sex organs.

CONFERENCE DEBATE

At one of the major political parties' national conferences some years ago three debates took place one morning, the first on agriculture and food production, the second on industry and efficient management and the third on the future of the Water Authorities.

In the third debate one representative, a doctor, started his contribution by saying: "I know nothing about agriculture and food production, I do not claim to be an expert in management and industry, but when it comes to water, I think I can hold my own!"

After a pause, while the comment sank in, it brought the house down.

conjugate deviation – a term describing persistent and involuntary turning of both eyes in any one direction; a sign of a lesion in the brain.

conjunctivitis – inflammation of the conjunctiva, the thin mucous membrane which covers the inside of the eyelids and the front of the eye. It may be the result of infection, allergy or irritation. It is sometimes known as 'pink eye'.

constipation – a condition whereby the bowels are opened too seldom or incompletely, giving rise to dry, hard motions.

consumption – another name for tuberculosis.

contact dermatitis – skin eruption, redness or inflammation due to contact with any of many materials or substances.

contracture – a permanent shortening of a muscle or fibrous tissue.

contre coup – an injury occurring not where the violence is applied, but on the opposite side – particularly in the skull.

contusion – bruising.

convulsion – an alternate contraction and relaxation of muscles causing irregular movements of the limbs of the body resulting from a disturbed function of the cerebral cortex; may be associated with frothing at the mouth, as in epilepsy; can occur in other conditions affecting the brain.

Cooley's anaemia – otherwise known as thalassaemia, a condition where there is an inherited defect in the production of normal haemoglobin.

coprolalia – a condition in which insane people shout filthy and obscene words.

coronary thrombosis – commonly called a heart attack whereby the coronary blood vessels, which supply blood to the heart muscle, become blocked either by a blood clot or due to constriction from chronic disease of the lining. Frequently it takes the form of acute constricting pain in the chest, like angina pectoris except that it does not go away.

corpulence – obesity.

cor pulmonale – a form of heart disease following chronic disease of the lungs. It culminates in failure of the right ventricle.

"Physicians of all men are most happy; what good success soever they have, the world proclaimeth, and what faults they commit the earth covereth".

Francis Quarles
(1592–1644)

Corrigan's pulse – collapsing pulse found in incompetence of the aortic valve (named after Dominic John Corrigan, 1802-1880, a famous Dublin physician).

coryza – another name for a cold in the head, caused by a virus infection. It is usually accompanied by blocking of the respiratory passages with mucus and catarrh and may be brought on by a draught or chill to the body surface, wetting of the feet or sudden immersion in water.

costalgia – pain in the ribs.

cot death – term applied to unexpected death of an apparently healthy baby (Sudden Infant Death Syndrome). Occurs in healthy or only slightly unwell infants, mostly aged 2–6 months, which are found dead in their cots, mostly occurring in bottle fed babies. It has been associated with placing the baby on its side or front, infection of the lungs, a bronchial virus or allergy to milk.

cough syncope – loss of consciousness induced by severe spasm of coughing.

cow pox – a disease affecting the udders of cows on which it produces vesicles; communicable to man, and persons who have caught it did not suffer from smallpox (this formed the basis of Jenner's experiments on smallpox vaccination).

coxa vara – a condition of the neck of the thigh bone, which is bent so that the lower limbs are turned outwards. Lameness ensues.

crabs – infestation by pubic lice.

cradle cap – patchy areas of greasy crusts on an infant's scalp due to the secretions of oil glands.

cramp – painful spasmodic contractions of muscles and sometimes some internal organs. Night cramps are most common, particularly in calf, foot and the back of the thigh. It also occurs in pregnancy. Cramp is common in athletes following extensive vigorous exercise due to the build up of lactic acid in the muscles with relative oxygen shortage.

creeping eruption – a skin condition caused by the larvae of certain nematode worms, which invade the skin leaving behind a long creeping red line.

cretinism – a disease due to defective thyroid function in foetal life and early pregnancy. The signs include feeding problems, constipation, failure and extreme sleepiness, apart from the facial appearance. If the diagnosis is delayed, numerous neurological abnormalities occur, along with abnormality of the gut, speech difficulties and, if not treated early, mental retardation may be permanent.

Creutzfeldt-Jakob disease – rapidly increasing dementia usually between the ages of 40-65, associated with other neurological signs; transmitted through a protein and believed to be associated with the agent causing 'mad cow disease' (BSE).

Crohn's disease – otherwise known as regional ileitis, it affects parts of the large intestine, but can affect any part of the gastrointestinal tract. Affected areas of the bowel become thickened and its lumen becomes narrowed due to extensive fibrosis. The patient suffers from repeated attacks of abdominal pain and chronic diarrhoea with bleeding. Complications can include intestinal adhesions and fistula formation.

croup – difficult laborious breathing with a cough in a child; caused by swelling and partial blockage of the entrance of the larynx. It can occur in acute laryngitis and diphtheria and can be dangerous; usually worse at night.

crush syndrome – kidney failure in patients who have been victims of a severe crush injury.

cryptococcosis – a rare disease due to infection with the yeast, Cryptococcus neoformans. It affects lungs, skin or meninges.

cryptorchidism – undescended testicle.

Cushing's syndrome – a disorder resulting from an excessive output of certain adrenal hormones. It is characterised by obesity, moon face, excess fat over the neck, shoulders and pelvis, purple striae, acne, increase in hair growth, a buffalo like hump and raised blood pressure.

HARVEY WILLIAM CUSHING was a leading American neurosurgeon of the early 20th century. He reduced the mortality rate associated with brain surgery and many of his techniques are still basic to this type of surgery.

His research on the pituitary in 1912 gained him an international reputation and he was the first to ascribe a type of obesity of the face (moonface) and the trunk, to pituitary malfunction.

This is now known as Cushing's disease or syndrome.

He won the Pullitzer prize in 1926 for his 'Life of William Ostler'.

Curling's ulcer – an ulcer of the stomach or duodenum associated with severe skin burns.

cyanosis – blueness about the face and extremities, including the lips and nose, due to the blood not being properly oxygenated.

cyclical oedema – irregular and intermittent bouts of general swelling due to fluid retention. It particularly occurs in women at the time of the menstrual period.

cycloplegia – paralysis of the ciliary muscle of the eye causing the loss of the ability of the eye to accommodate.

cyesis – another name for pregnancy.

cystic fibrosis – most commonly seen genetic disease in caucasian children (1:2000); a disorder of the mucous secreting glands of the lungs, pancreas, mouth and gastrointestinal tract. The infant fails to thrive, suffers from repeated attacks of bronchitis and produces foul smelling and slimy stools. Regular treatment with physiotherapy is required along with the administration of pancreatic enzymes. Twenty years ago only 12% survived into adulthood, now 75% survive into their forties.

cystitis – inflammation of the bladder, most commonly due to infection by the bacteria which normally inhabit the bowel. The condition is more common in women and gives rise to burning or stinging pain on passing water, frequency of passing water, and sometimes the presence of blood in the urine.

cyst – a hollow sac or cavity containing liquids or semi-solid material. It is almost always benign.

cysticercosis – infestation of the body with larvae of the tapeworm.

dacrocystitis – a condition whereby the lacrimal sac (sac containing tears) becomes inflamed. Infection usually arises in the nose and throat and appears as a tender swelling at the medial angle of the eyes.

dactylitis – inflammation of the finger or toe.

dandruff – fine, whitish, greasy scales formed upon the scalp (seborrhoea).

day blindness – a patient sees better in dim light or at night; usually brought on by being in glaring light e.g. in the desert or snow.

deafness – a defect in hearing or the inability to hear at all. It can occur due to an abnormality of any of the three parts of the ear; the outer ear, usually due to a blockage e.g. wax or infection; the middle ear due to infection of the inner ear and brain due to a variety of conditions e.g. senile deafness. There are two specific types; conductive deafness, an interruption in the transmission of sound, and perceptive deafness, which implies auditory nerve (VIIIth cranial nerve) deficiency.

debility – a state of weakness.

decompensation – a failing condition of the heart in cases of valvular disease.

decubitus – the name of peculiar positions taken up in bed by patients suffering from different conditions. Hence bedsores are known as decubitus ulcers.

deficiency disease – a disease resulting from absence from the diet of any substance essential to good health e.g. vitamins.

deformities – may be present at birth, the result of injuries or disease or simply produced by bad habits e.g. the curved spine sometimes found in children.

degeneration – a change in structure or in chemical composition of a tissue or organ where vitality is lowered or function interfered with. Apart from specific forms of degeneration (like fatty) it may simply be due to disease or old age.

déjà vu – an illusion that a present experience has occurred before.

Delhi boil – a chronic sore occurring in eastern countries caused by the protozoan parasite, Leishmania tropica.

delirium – a condition of altered consciousness in which there is disorientation, incoherent talk, restlessness with hallucinations, illusions or delusions. In elderly people it is often referred to as confusion.

delirium tremens – a form of delirium most commonly due to the sudden withdrawal of alcohol if the person has become dependent on it. It presents as restlessness, fear or even terror usually accompanied by vivid visual hallucinations (traditional 'pink elephants', insects crawling all over the person, rats etc.), and disorientation of time, place or person.

delusion – a false belief to which the patient adheres despite firm evidence to the contrary.

dementia – a general term for mental deterioration, usually including serious impairment of intellect, irrationality, confusion and insane behaviour. It may result from physical changes in the brain, poisons, toxins produced by disease or psychoses.

De Morgan spots – small haemangiomas (benign tumour composed of a conglomeration of dilated small blood vessels) in the skin of middle aged people, which are of no clinical significance.

dengue – sudden fever with severe pain in the muscles and joints (breakbone fever), due to an arbovirus transmitted by the mosquito Aedes aegypti; also accompanied by skin eruptions. It is not a dangerous disease and the patient recovers spontaneously.

depression – a mental condition characterised by the sufferer being in a state of melancholy and gloom, sometimes accompanied by a feeling of inadequacy and a lack of energy.

DeQuervains's disease – a thickening of the sheaths covering the tendons of the thumb, giving rise to pain at its base, which radiates to the nail and into the forearm.

Derbyshire neck – another name for a type of goitre; so named because it was common in a part of Derbyshire where there was a shortage of iodine in the drinking water.

dermagraphia – condition in which tracings on the skin leave a distinct reddish mark. It occurs in allergic individuals in whom scratching of the skin produces excessive amounts of histamine.

dermatitis – inflammation of the skin, similar to eczema; types include contact, light and exfoliative. The condition starts with patches of erythema (redness) and can extend to involve the whole body. Eventually patches of the skin start to peel.

dermatitis herpetiformis – small blisters appearing mainly on the convex surfaces of the body; an immunological condition due to sensitivity to gluten.

dermatomyositis – an auto-immune disease with erythema of the skin and wasting of the muscles. It also presents with inflammation of the skin of the face, upper trunk and extremities.

dermatophytosis – fungal infections of the skin e.g. athlete's foot, scalp ringworm, tinea corporis and nail infections.

dermoid cyst – a congenital cyst which contains fragments of skin appendages, such as hairs, sweat glands, cartilage, bone and teeth.

desquamation – scaling off of the superficial layer of the skin.

deviated septum – a deviation from a straight line of the wall that divides the nose into two equal parts, usually as a result of injury. It may lead to partial obstruction of the air passages.

Devonshire colic – a condition caused by drinking cider which has been standing in contact with lead. The colic is due to lead poisoning.

> **dextrocardia** – a congenital condition in which the axis of the heart has been transposed to the right side of the chest.

Dhobi itch – see tinea cruris.

diabetes insipidus – a condition in which there is excessive thirst with the passing of a large amount of urine; either due to lack of the anti-diuretic hormone (ADH), normally produced in the hypothalamus and stored in the posterior pituitary gland, or a defect in the renal tubules, which prevents them responding to ADH.

diabetes mellitus – due to a defect in the production of the hormone insulin by the pancreas. Characterised by the presence of a high blood sugar and the presence of sugar in the urine (glycosuria). There are two types, type 1 or insulin dependent, in which the condition requires insulin injections and type 2, usually due to obesity and developing in later life. The latter type can be controlled by diet and/or oral medication. Untreated, diabetes proceeds to ketosis, coma and death.

> In 1921 Charles Best, while still an undergraduate, became a laboratory assistant to the physician Frederick Banting in the laboratory of the physiologist J J R Macleod at the University of Toronto. In the same year they were able to isolate the hormone insulin, which they found would control diabetes in dogs. The hormone was subsequently found to be as effective in humans.
> In 1923 Banting, as head of the department of medical research, received the Nobel prize for physiology and medicine together with Macleod. As Best did not receive his Doctor of Medicine degree until 1925 he did not share the prize.
> Banting was killed in a plane crash on a war mission in 1941, while Best, who succeeded Banting as Director of the Banting and Best Department of Medical Research, became the first to introduce anticoagulants in the treatment of thrombosis.

diaphoresis – another name for sweating.

diarrhoea – abnormal frequency and looseness of stools. In young infants it can cause serious loss of fluids and electrolytes.

> "The healthy stomach is nothing if not conservative. Few radicals have good digestions"
> Samuel Butler (1835-1902)

diastasis – separation of the end of a growing bone from its shaft.

dicephalus – foetal 'monster' having two heads.

dicrotic pulse – at each heartbeat two impulses can be felt by the fingers.

Dietl's crisis – occurs in those who have mobile kidneys, where there is kinking of the ureter producing attacks of intense abdominal pain radiating down the ureter with nausea, vomiting, fever and collapse. If it is accompanied by hydronephrosis, surgery may be necessary.

digitalis poisoning – occurs when digitalis (medicine prepared from foxglove) is taken over too long a period or when a single overdose is taken; characterised by nausea and vomiting, blurring of vision, with objects appearing yellow or green. After being slowed, the heart quickens and becomes irregular, breathing becomes difficult. Convulsions or unconsciousness follow.

diphtheria – an acute infectious disease characterised by a membranous exudate on the mucous surfaces of the tonsils, the back of the throat and larynx, due to the bacterium Corynebacterium diphtheriae. The general symptoms are due to the absorption of a toxin which can cause damage to the heart muscle. It is highly infectious with an incubation period of 2–6 days. In serious cases a membrane can cause obstruction of the larynx. It can be treated with antitoxin and antibiotics. While the disease can be prevented by mass inoculation programmes, any relaxation of this policy could result in the return of epidemics of this potentially fatal disease.

Diphtheria sometimes referred to as 'angina maligna' has been around for some time.
In 1659 the preacher Cotton Mather reported that 'a malady of bladder in the windpipe' killed a number of children in the Massachusetts Bay colony.
George Washington died at Mount Vernon on December 15th 1799 of asphyxia from a severely swollen throat.
The description of his last illness makes a diphtheria diagnosis virtually certain.
The former American President was probably the most famous adult victim of the disease.

Diphyllobothrium latum – a fish tapeworm giving rise to a type of megaloblastic anaemia.

diplegia – paralysis affecting both sides of the body severely.

diplopia – double vision.

diprosopus – a foetus which has two faces instead of one.

dipsomania – a morbid and insatiable craving for alcohol.

dipygus – a foetus with a double pelvis.

discharge – abnormal emission from any part of the body.

dislocation – the displacement of a bone from its normal position in a joint usually the result in a blow, fall or twisting force.

disorientation – a lack of awareness of time and place in the relation to self and the environment.

distichiasis – a term applied to a condition in which there are two complete rows of eyelids on each side.

diverticulitis – inflammation of the diverticuli of the large intestine. The diverticuli are pouches or pockets leading off the main cavity or tube; otherwise a protrusion from the intestine. Where there is no inflammation, the condition is known as diverticulosis.

dizziness – a feeling of unsteadiness and of everything revolving around. It can be due to a disturbance in the inner ear, a reduced blood supply to the brain or many other conditions. Not usually a symptom of serious disease but recurrent attacks should be investigated.

Down's syndrome – a congenital condition which is sometimes referred to as 'mongolism' due to the mongoloid features of those with the condition. The cause is the presence of an extra chromosome, 47 instead of 46, in the cells of the individual; often associated with other congenital abnormalities such as heart conditions, resulting in a low life expectation in a number with the syndrome. The condition is more common in infants of more elderly mothers. There are varying degrees of mental subnormality, but most of those who survive can learn to carry out simple work and some 5% can learn to read.

dracunculiasis – a disease caused by the guinea worm, Dracunculus mediensis. It is transmitted by cyclops, a fresh water crustacean and man is infested by drinking contaminated water. It causes no trouble for the first year of infection but the worm works through to the surface of the body causing a painful swelling and fever. It may be necessary to remove the worm surgically although the condition can be treated by chemotherapy. The female worm can grow to up to 4 feet long. It is believed to be the mosaic 'fiery serpent' that harassed the Israelites on the shore of the Red Sea. It occurs in tropical Africa and Asia.

drepanocytosis – another name for sickle cell anaemia.

drop attacks – usually occurs in middle aged women when the legs suddenly give way and the sufferer falls to the ground without warning but with no loss of consciousness; no obvious cause but it is thought that there may be temporary interference with the blood supply to the brain or, in a small number of cases, a vestibular effect. Recovery is usually immediate.

drop foot – there is difficulty in raising the front part of the foot from the ground or the foot hangs limp, due to neuritis in the nerves supplying the muscle on the front of the leg.

dropped beat – means the missing out of a regular heart beat; may be due to heart block or as compensation for an extra heart beat.

dropsy – another name for oedema.

William Withering (1741–1799) was both a Physician and Botanist. He obtained his MD at Edinburgh in 1766 and was elected FRS in 1785. After being appointed as Physician to the County Infirmary Stafford in 1767 he moved on to the Birmingham General Hospital in 1775. Withering was the first to use digitalis on a patient on hearing that the foxglove was good for the dropsy from an old country woman. He published "An Account of the Foxglove" in 1776.

drop wrist – complete or partial paralysis of muscles which extend the hand; one of the causes is known as 'crutch palsy', where the head of a crutch presses on the nerve plexus in the axilla (armpit). It can also be caused by the person sleeping with the head resting on the upper arm or the arm over the back of the chair

drug interaction – a condition whereby drugs which may be free of adverse effects when given individually, produce severe adverse effects when given together.

ductus arteriosus – a blood vessel in the foetus through which blood passes from the pulmonary artery into the aorta, bypassing the lungs which do not function in utero. The vessel ceases to function soon after birth and closes up leaving a fibrous cord. If obliteration does not occur it results in a condition known as 'patent ductus arteriosus'. This is the most common congenital defect of the heart.

dumbness – inability to pronounce the sounds which go to make up words; usually associated with deafness. If hearing is normal it may be due to mental deficiency.

dumping syndrome – symptoms of abdominal distention, diarrhoea and vomiting, occurring soon after eating in those who have had their stomachs partially removed.

duodenal ileus – dilatation of the duodum due to some chronic obstruction caused by the abnormal positioning of an artery near the duodenum and pressing on it.

duodenal ulcer – a type of peptic ulcer, more common than a gastric ulcer and less likely to become malignant.

The cause is unknown, but there is usually some abrasion in the mucous membrane, which becomes eroded and deepened by the gastric juice.

It can be made worse by stress, smoking and alcohol; pain tends to occur 2-3 hours after a meal and relieved by food and antacids; complications include perforation or bleeding.

Dupuytren's contracture – a thickening of the skin and connective tissue of the palm of the hand, pulling one or more fingers down. It usually affects the little and ring fingers first.

THE ROYAL SURGEON

Baron Guillaume Dupuytren (1777-1835) must have been an extremely versatile surgeon. Apart from describing and developing surgical procedures to alleviate the contracture that bears his name in 1832, he had also been the first surgeon to excise the lower jaw (1812) and to provide the first clear description of congenital dislocation of the hip (1826). The Baron also introduced a new classification of burns, carried out surgery for carcinoma of the cervix, the creation of an artificial anus (1828), ligation of the subclavian artery, treated aneurysms by compression and surgically treated cases of wry neck.

He was surgeon to Louis XVIII, who created him a Baron, and to Charles X.

dwarfism – a term applied to underdevelopment of the body, either a developmental condition or due to food insufficiency. The commonest type is pituitary dwarfism caused by deficiency in the production of growth hormone secreted by the anterior pituitary. All parts develop in normal proportion to each other but overall small in size. It can be treated by administering growth hormone to children. Dwarfism can also be due to rickets early in life.

dysarthria – due to a weakness or incoordination of the muscles of speech, producing a slurring and weakness of speech, usually caused by damage affecting speech centres in the brain or the muscles themselves; present following strokes, cerebral palsy, Parkinson's disease, multiple sclerosis and motor neurone disease.

dyschezia – constipation due to the retention of faeces in the rectum; the outcome of irregular bowel habits.

dyscrasia – an abnormal state particularly of the blood.

dysdiokokinesia – the loss of ability to perform rapid alternate movements e.g. winding up a watch; a sign of abnormality in the cerebellum.

dysentery – inflammation of the colon with severe diarrhoea, abdominal cramps and sometimes blood and mucus in the stools (the bloody flux). There are two major forms, bacillary, occurring anywhere in the world, or amoebic, occurring in the tropical or subtropical regions.

dysidrosis – a disturbance of sweat secretion.

dyslexia – difficulty in reading or learning to read, accompanied by difficulty in writing or spelling. It may be caused by defective vision, mental backwardness, psychological causes or the effects of physical disease. There is also the specific form of the condition where it occurs in an otherwise normal and intelligent person. It is three times more common in boys and is sometimes referred to as 'word blindness'.

dysmenhorroea – painful menstruation.

dyspareunia – pain experienced by women during intercourse.

dyspepsia – another name for indigestion.

dysphagia – difficulty in swallowing.

dysphasia – difficulty in understanding languages or in self-expression. It often occurs after a stroke or other brain damage.

dyspnoea – difficulty in breathing.

dystonia – a type of involuntary movement due to sustained muscle contraction, twisting and repetitive movements or abnormal postures, as a result of inappropriate instructions coming from the brain.

dystrophia – defective or faulty nutrition. It is also a term generally applied to some developmental change in the muscles occurring independently of the nervous system. The best known form is progressive muscular dystrophy where the muscles undergo fatty degeneration and will increase in size but with a weakness in power.

dysuria – difficulty or pain on passing water.

ebola virus disease – viral haemorrhagic fever.

ecchyma – pustular eruption with surrounding inflammation. After the pustule has discharged, a pigmented scar is left.

ecchymosis – discoloured patches resulting from the escape of blood into the tissues just under the skin.

> **echolalia** – meaningless repetition, by a person suffering from mental degeneration, of words and phrases addressed to him or her.

echinococcus – immature form of small tapeworm found in dogs, jackals and wolves. When humans become infected it takes the form of hydatid disease with the formation hydatid cysts.

eclampsia – a serious form of convulsions occurring in late pregnancy or during and after delivery. It is an extreme manifestation of toxaemia of pregnancy.

ecstasy – a morbid mental condition where the mind is entirely absorbed with one idea or object and loses the sense of time and self control. It often presents as religious insanity.

ectopic – means out of place, as in ectopic testis and ectopic pregnancy.

ectromelia – absence of a limb or limbs from congenital causes.

ectropion – the eye lid turns outwards – more commonly in the lower than upper lid.

eczema – a general term for inflammation of the skin; usually the reaction of the skin to a wide range of stimulants or irritants.

effort syndrome – palpitations and shortness of breath attributed by the patient to a disorder of the heart, with no clinical sign of heart disease. Otherwise known as Da Costa's syndrome.

effusion – pouring out of fluid from vessels in which it is normally contained into the substance of an organ or into the body cavity, as a result of inflammation or injury e.g. pleural effusion in the thoracic cavity.

electric injuries – usually caused by the passage of an electric current through the body.

elephantiasis – a disease characterised by gross overgrowth of skin and the tissue spaces underneath. It is seen in tropical countries in those suffering from the effects of the parasite Filaria bancrofti which blocks the lymphatic vessels. It particularly affects the legs and scrotum.

emaciation – pronounced wasting.

embolism – the obstruction of a blood vessel by an embolus which consists of material carried by the blood stream e.g. a clot, a mass of bacteria, air bubble. It can cause the destruction of an organ or part of an organ supplied by that blood vessel.

emesis – a term for vomiting.

emphysema – the abnormal presence of air in a part of the body. It normally refers to a condition of the lungs characterised by over distension of the air sacs.

emprosthotonos – a spasm of the belly muscle occurring in tetanus making the body arch forwards.

empyema – the accumulation of pus within a cavity. It usually refers to the pleural cavity (as a complication of lobar pneumonia).

encephalitis – inflammation of the brain usually due to a virus. It is sometimes a complication of a common infectious disease such as measles and mumps.

encephaloid – a form of cancer which resembles brain tissue to the naked eye.

encephalomyelitis – inflammation of the substance of the brain and spinal cord.

encephalopathy – describes certain conditions in which there are signs of cerebral irritation, without any localised lesion to account for it. It can occur in the later stage of kidney disease or uraemia – giving rise to hypertensive encephalopathy with convulsions and delirium.

enchondroma – a tumour formed from cartilage.

endarteritis – inflammation of the inner part of an artery.

endocarditis – inflammation of the smooth membrane lining the heart, particularly the heart valves.

endometriosis – endometrium found in parts of the body other than that lining the uterus, e.g. the muscle of the uterus.

endometritis – inflammation of the mucous lining of the uterus.

enophthalmos – abnormal retraction of eye into the socket.

enteralgia – another name for colic.

enteric fever – typhoid or paratyphoid fever.

enteritis – inflammation of the intestine.

enterobiasis – infestation with Enterobius vermicularis or thread worm, the most common intestinal parasite in the U.K. They cause irritation around the anus and scratching can help to reinfect by reingestion of the eggs from the fingers.

enteroptosis – a lax condition of the mesentery, which causes the bowel to drop into the lower half of the abdomen.

enterostomy – an operation to make an artificial opening into the intestine.

entomophobia – an excessive fear of insects particularly spiders.

entropion – the eye lid turns inwards, particularly the lower lids.

enuresis – unconscious or involuntary passage of urine.

> **eosinophilia** – an abnormal increase in the number of eosinophils (a type of white blood cell). It occurs in Hodgkin's disease, asthma, hay fever, skin disease and parasite infestation.

ephelis – a freckle.

epiglottitis – inflammation of the epiglottis. The acute variety is usually due to the bacteria Haemophilus influenzae, a serious condition in children where the epiglottis becomes swollen, obstructing the air passage. It can be fatal.

epignathus – a mal development of the foetus, whereby the deformed remnant of one twin becomes united with the upper jaw of the other.

epilepsy – any of various brain disorders characterised by sudden recurring attacks of motor, sensory or psychic malfunction with or without unconsciousness or convulsive movements. There are two principle types: primary epilepsy where there is no known cause and secondary epilepsy, which is secondary to some known disease e.g. cerebral tumour.

epistaxis – bleeding from the nose.

epithelioma – a malignant tumour arising from the epithelium covering the outside of the body.

epulis – any tumour of the jaw.

Erb's paralysis – any paralysis of the arm due to stretching or tearing of the nerves of the brachial plexus. This may occur due to injury during childbirth. The paralysis takes the form of the arm dropping down next to the adjacent side with the elbow extended and the forearm pronated in the so called 'waiter's tip' position.

erethism – chronic mercurial poisoning giving rise to irritability, self-consciousness, timidity, lack of concentration, depression and resenting criticism. The condition used to be an occupational hazard in the hat industry, (mercury was used in felt hat production) – hence 'as mad as a hatter'.

ergotism – due to ergot poisoning. There is intense pain with hallucinations along with spasmodic contraction of the muscles and gangrene of the fingers, tips of the ears and toes. It is due to spasmodic constriction of the blood vessels. The condition could occur as a consequence of eating bread made with diseased rye.

erosion – the process of the gradual wearing down of structures of the body.

eructation – belching. The escape of gas or portions of half digested food from the body of the stomach into the mouth. It can cause acid dyspepsia.

eruption – an outburst in scattered form on the surface of the skin usually raised and red, but it may consist of scales, crusts or vesicles; in other words a rash.

erysipelis – an acute bacterial infection of the skin and underlying tissue, accompanied by a fever. The infection is caused by Strepococcus pyogenes. It is slightly more common in women than men and is sometimes known as St.Anthony's fire. It can occur just after delivery in women. A rare acute serious form occurs in the newborn, erisepalis neonatorum. As with all strepococcal infections, the condition responds to treatment with penicillin.

erythema – redness of the skin.

erythrasma – a reddish brown macular eruption of the skin due to the micro-organism Nocardia minutissima.

erythroblastosis – a disease of newborn infants associated with rhesus incompatibility of the mother and child.

erythroedema – a disease of infants characterised by weakness, neuritis, swelling and redness of the face, fingers and toes. It is usually due to mercurial poisoning, possibly from teething powders. Another name is 'pink disease'.

erythromelalgia – a condition in which the fingers, toes and even large portions of the limbs become purple and bloated. It is worse in the summer when parts are allowed to hang down. Sometimes the condition has no known cause or it can be associated with vascular disease or metallic poisoning; otherwise known as 'red neuralgia'.

> **essential hypertension** – the most common form of high blood pressure. The cause is not known.

exanthemata – the old name used to classify the acute infectious disease, which is associated with a rash.

exfoliation – a separation in layers of pieces of dead bone or skin.

exomphalos – a hernia formed by the projection of the abdominal organs through the umbilicus.

exophthalmos – bulging eyes, a condition characteristic of some forms of thyroid disease, such as exophthalmic goitre.

exostosis – an outgrowth from a bone.

expectoration – the bringing up of material, such as sputum, from the chest or air passages.

exstrophy of the bladder – a congenital malformation of the bladder in which it has no abdominal covering and the urine comes out on to the surface of the body.

extrasystole – premature contraction of one or more chambers of the heart, when the beat occurs sooner than it should followed by a compensating pause.

extravasation – the escape of fluid from the vessels or passages which ought to contain it e.g. the bladder, when the bladder or urethra rupture.

exudation – some constituents of the blood pass through the walls of the small vessels in the course of inflammation, also the accumulation resulting from the process e.g. the solid rough material deposited on the surface of the lung in pleurisy. Exudation is the term also applied to the process of sweating.

fainting – temporary loss of consciousness most often caused by a temporary inadequate supply of blood reaching the brain e.g. standing up suddenly from the lying or sitting position; otherwise known as syncope.

falling sickness – another name for epilepsy.

Fanconi's syndrome – multiple inherited abnormalities which impair kidney function and depress blood cell formation in the bone marrow.

farcy – another name for glanders.

farmer's lung – a form of allergic alveolitis due to the inhalation of dust from mouldy hay or straw.

fasciitis – inflammation of the fascia; the commonest site is in the sole of the foot (see policeman's heel).

fascioliasis – disease caused by the liver fluke, Fasciola hepatica. The symptoms include fever, dyspepsia, sweating, loss of appetite, abdominal pain, urticaria and troublesome cough. It can be transmitted from the eggs of the fluke by eating wild watercress. Passed from animals to man by the snail.

fastigium – the highest temperature reached in a feverish state.

fat necrosis – occurs following inflammation or injury to the pancreas, after which fat splitting enzymes may escape.

fatty degeneration – takes place as a result of anaemia which interferes with the blood supply or nerve supply or because of the action of various poisons e.g. alcohol. The body cells undergo many abnormal changes accompanied by the appearance of fat droplets in their substance.

favism – a haemolytic anaemia from eating broad beans; an hereditary condition due to the lack of glucose-6-phosphate dehydrogenase. It is present in 14% of American negroes and 60% of Yemenite Jews in Israel.

favus – another name for honeycomb ringworm.

fester – a popular term used to mean any collection or formation of pus.

Felty's syndrome – a chronic arthritis with enlargement of the spleen and a decrease in a certain type of white blood cells.

fetishism – a form of sexual deviation in which the person becomes sexually stimulated by parts of the body such as the feet which are not usually erotogenic.

fever – a condition characterised by a rise in temperature.

> **fibrillation** – a term applied to the rapid contraction or tremor of muscles, especially to the form of abnormal action of the heart muscle in which the individual bundles of fibres take up an independent action.

fibrocystic disease of the pancreas – see cystic fibrosis.

fibroid – a term applied to a tumour of the womb which is part muscular and part fibrous tissue.

fibroma – a tumour consisting of fibrous tissue.

fibrosis – the formation of fibrous or scar tissue due either to infection or a deficiency of the blood supply.

fibrositis – another name for muscular rheumatism.

fibrous dysplasia – a rare disease in which areas of the bone are replaced by fibrous tissue leaving the bones fragile and likely to fracture.

> **filariasis** – the name given to a group of tropical diseases in which the nematode worms (filaria) are found in the blood; the most common is Filarium bancrofti or Wucheria bancrofti. The adult female can grow to 100mm in length. It occurs in Sri Lanka, SE Asia, China, New Guinea, Tropical Africa. (see elephantiasis).

fissure – a break or crack in the skin or a membrane; most frequent in the rectal area.

fistula – an abnormal channel between body parts or leading from a hollow organ to a free surface, usually discharging fluid or material from an organ.

fit – another name for a sudden convulsive seizure.

flat foot – a deformity of the foot in which the arch sinks down and the inner edge of the foot comes to rest on the ground (pes planus).

flatulence – a collection of gas in the stomach or bowels.

flexibilitas cerea – an abnormal state in which the limbs remain in any position in which they are moved.

floaters – cells or strands of tissue which float in the vitreous humour of the eye and move with the movement of the eyeball, casting shadows on the retina. They look like small spots and are more annoying than serious.

floating kidney – a kidney which is abnormally movable from its normal place because it is loosely attached and is poorly supported by surrounding fat. There is a slightly higher risk of developing some kidney conditions such as hydronephrosis and Dietl's crisis.

floccitation – fitful picking at the bedclothes by a delirious patient.

flooding – popular name for excess bleeding from the womb, particularly during a heavy period. It can be a sign of a miscarriage.

flukes – parasitic flatworms which cause infestation of the intestines, liver and lungs.

fluoridism – caused by excess intake of fluoride giving rise to such signs as mottling of the teeth. Occurs in very hot and dry regions where the fluoride level in the water is excessively high.

flutter – term given to a form of abnormal cardiac rhythm.

flux – excessive discharge from any of the natural openings of the body.

folie à deux – a form of mental disorder usually in two close friends who both have the same delusions e.g. the two old ladies in the play 'Arsenic and Old Lace'.

food intolerance – a condition, usually psychological, in which the person has an inability to eat certain foods. Only rarely is this due to a specific food allergy.

food poisoning – due to eating contaminated food which is either contaminated with chemical or metallic poisons, bacteria or toxins produced by them.

foot drop – dropping of the feet due to the paralysis of the muscles or tendons that extend or lift it.

fractures – breaches in the structure of bones produced by violence.

framboesia – another name for yaws.

> **Friedrich's ataxia** – an hereditary disease resembling locomotor ataxia. It is a degenerative disease affecting the nerve tracts and usually occurs in children or those under twenty. The condition manifests itself with unsteadiness of gait, loss of knee jerks, difficulty in speech, tremors of the body, head and eyes, deformity of the feet and curvature of the spine. It can last for 20–30 years with gradual deterioration.

frigidity – sexual coldness in women. More often it is of psychological origin, but there can be some physical cause.

Froehlich's syndrome – a condition in children characterised by obesity, sluggishness and retarded sexual development. The condition is the result of impairment of the functions of the pituitary and thymus glands. (like the fat boy in Dickens' Pickwick Papers).

frostbite – a condition due to exposure to severe cold. The extremities become white and numb, the part becoming 'dead' followed by pain. Blisters frequently occur and, in severe cases, gangrene.

frozen shoulder – a painful condition of the shoulder accompanied by stiffness and limitation of the movement.

> **fugue** – used to describe a mental condition where the individual is suddenly seized with an unconscious desire to flee from the intolerable reality of everyday existence. It lasts for a matter of hours or days, with an odd manner of behaviour which may be put down to eccentricity. There is no remembrance of events afterwards.

functional disease – another name for psychosomatic disease.

funnel chest – a congenital deformity in which the breastbone is depressed towards the spine, forming a funnel shaped cavity (pectus excavatum).

furfuraceous – a term applied to disease which produce scaliness of the skin.

furuncle – another name for a boil.

galactocoele – a cyst like swelling in the breast as a result of obstruction of a milk duct draining the swollen area.

galactorrhoea – a recurrent or persistent discharge of milk from the breast.

galactosaemia – an hereditary condition of infants who cannot digest milk, due to the lack of enzyme which converts galactose (the sugar derived from lactose) into glucose. Unless all milk products are removed from the diet, toxic accumulation of galactose in the blood leads to damage to the lens of the eye, brain and kidney. Cataracts and mental retardation can also occur.

GALENICALS

Galen classified thousands of plant materials around 150 AD and concocted numerous prescriptions.
To this day medicines prepared from vegetable sources to standard formulae are sometimes known as 'galenicals'.

gallop rhythm – sounds of the heart resembling the gallop of a horse, indicating a failing heart muscle.

gallstones – stones formed in the gallbladder or its ducts due either to stasis, increased concentration or infection. They may or may not cause symptoms.

ganglion – a name given to a cyst of a tendon sheath, usually on the back or front of the wrist. Anatomically a ganglion is also the name given to a cluster of nerve cells.

gangrene – death of tissue due to a failure of the blood supply to an area. May be due to many causes e.g. diseased blood vessels, frostbite, burns, crush injury, pressure on or obstruction of the blood vessels. It may be wet or dry, wet gangrene occurring when infection is superimposed upon the gangrene giving rise to an offensive watery discharge. Diabetics are especially prone to gangrene.

gargoylism – an hereditary condition in children characterised by protruding abdomen, large head, short arms and legs, mental deficiency and opacities in the cornea. The condition is due to the lack of a specific enzyme and is a progressive disease leading to death before the age of ten (Hurler's syndrome).

gas gangrene – a serious infection of the injured tissue caused by the spore bearing bacteria Clostridium welchii, which produces bubbles of foul smelling gas.

gastralgia – pain in the stomach.

gastric ulcer – a type of peptic ulcer occurring in the stomach usually adjacent to the acid producing section. It is more likely to become malignant than a duodenal ulcer, but this is still a rare complication. Other complications include haemorrhage and perforation. More common in men than women. Both gastric and duodenal ulcers are more common in those with the blood group O.

gastritis – inflammation of the stomach.

gastroenteritis – inflammation of the stomach and intestine usually giving rise to diarrhoea and vomiting.

> "He healeth those that are broken in heart; and giveth medicine to heal their sickness."
> From the 1662 Prayer Book

gastroenterostomy – an artificial opening, produced surgically, between the stomach and small intestine, usually made to bypass an obstruction in the stomach e.g. tumour.

gastroptosis – a condition in which the stomach occupies an abnormally low point in the abdomen.

gastrostomy – an opening made into the front of the stomach so that fluid can be passed directly in, necessary due to a blockage in the gullet.

gathering – term applied to an abscess.

Gaucher's disease – an hereditary disorder of fat metabolism. It is characterised by an enlargement of the spleen and liver, associated with bone and joint pains and brown pigmentation of the skin due to accumulation of fat like substances.

general paralysis of the insane – a degeneration of bodily and mental powers, sometimes associated with delusions of grandeur and pupil signs. A late manifestation of tertiary syphilis (GPI).

genu valgum – medical term for knock knees.

genu varum – medical term for bow legs.

German measles – otherwise known as rubella; an acute virus disease, mild in nature and accompanied by slight fever, a pink rash with swelling of the glands of the neck. If the condition occurs in the early stages of pregnancy it may be responsible for congenital defects of the foetus.

giardiasis – a condition caused by the parasite Giardia lamblia. The condition is often harmless but it may give rise to diarrhoea with pale fatty stools. There are usually about 3000 cases a year reported in the U.K., usually caused by drinking untreated water in the Middle East or Russia.

gigantism – see acromegaly.

giggle micturition – a sudden involuntary complete emptying of the bladder during laughter, as opposed to just dampening of the pants.

gingivitis – inflammation of the gums.

glanders – a contagious often chronic and fatal disease of horses and other similar animals such as asses and mules. It is caused by the bacterium Loefflerella mallei and is characterised by a nasal discharge and ulcers in the lungs, respiratory tract and the skin. It occasionally can be passed on to man, usually those who work with horses. It has largely been eradicated from the U.K., but it still occurs in Eastern Europe and Asia.

glandular fever – otherwise known as infectious mononucleosis. It is a virus infection usually affecting older children, adolescents and young adults. It is characterised by fever, sore throat, enlarged glands in the neck and sometimes enlarged spleen and jaundice. There is also a chronic loss of appetite. Blood examinations shows an increase in the mononuclear white blood cells. A specific test, the Paul Bunnell test is usually positive. In adults convalescence may be prolonged.

glaucoma – a condition of the eye whereby the pressure of the fluid in the eye is raised. In an acute form it may come on suddenly causing acute pain. It can cause damage to the nervous plexus in the eye and the optic nerve leading to blindness.

gleet – a chronic form of gonorrhoea.

glioma – a tumour found in the brain and spinal cord affecting the neuroglia, a special connective tissue in those organs supporting the nerve cells and nerve fibres.

glomerulonephritis – an acute or chronic inflammation of the fine blood vessels in the glomerulus of the kidney. It is usually bilateral and may be due to an auto–immune response.

glossitis – inflammation of the tongue.

glue ear – another name for otitis media when thick secretions are present.

glycogen storage disease – an hereditary disorder of infants. There is a lack of certain enzymes necessary for glucose metabolism, leading to abnormal deposits of glycogen in various tissues of the body with slowing down of the bodily processes.

glycosuria – the presence of sugar in the urine.

goitre – a term applied to a swelling in the front of the neck due to enlargement of the thyroid gland.

golfer's elbow – similar to tennis elbow; an inflammation in the tendons on the muscles that extend or straighten the elbow.

gonagra – an attack of gout affecting the knee.

gonorrhoea – a venereal infection caused by the bacterium Neisseria gonorrhoeae. The infection affects the urethra in the male and the vagina in the female producing irritation and yellowish discharge. The infection can spread upwards to affect other parts of the urogenital system. Treatment is with penicillin and other antibiotics.

STUDENT WIT

Wit, sometimes of the classical variety, is never in short supply when medical students are around.

In the Medical School of one of the London Teaching Hospitals it was the usual practice to have the day's operating list pinned on the notice board.

This occasionally included the odd secretarial mis-spelling.

One day on the list was written "Removal of **Gaul** Bladder." A student had written underneath "In Trés Partes?"

gout – a constitutional disorder of metabolism producing an excess of uric acid in the blood stream and crystals become deposited in the joints. This can give rise to acute inflammation in the affected joints causing severe pain. The commonest joint to be affected is in the big toe. It can also be caused by the administration of certain diuretic drugs which diminish the normal excretion of uric acid.

grand mal – a convulsive epileptic attack.

granular kidney – chronic glomerulonephritis associated with chronic arteriosclerosis of the kidney.

granuloma – tumour or new growth in tissue made up of granular tissue. Can be caused by various forms of chronic inflammation such as TB or syphilis.

granuloma inguinale – a mildly contagious venereal disease produced by the bacterium Donovana granulomatosis. Granulomatous swellings occur in the inguinal, genital and perineal regions with ulceration and scarring.

Graves' disease – characterised by goitre, hyperthyroidism and exophthalmos; another name for exophthalmic goitre.

Green's sickness – another name for chlorosis.

greenstick fracture – an incomplete fracture occurring when the bone is not broken right across. It occurs mainly in children.

grinders' rot – a disease of the lungs in steel grinders caused by inhaling particles of the metal.

gripes – another name for colic in infants.

grippe – popular name for influenza.

growth – another name for tumour.

gumboil – inflammation generally ending up as an abscess in the root of a careous tooth.

gumma – hard swelling usually in connective tissue, internal organs, muscle, brain or skin. It is usually painless and is manifestation of tertiary syphilis.

gynaecomastia – an abnormal increase in the size of the male breast.

habit spasm – occurs in any individual of any occupation or handicraft. It is due to overactivity of the part concerned; e.g. wry neck through following some activity with the head.

haemangioma – a benign tumour made up of tortuous blood vessels.

haemarthrosis – bleeding into a joint.

haematemesis – the vomiting of blood; usually a complication of peptic ulceration, cancer of the stomach, gastritis or ruptured oesophageal varices.

haematocoele – a cavity containing blood. It occurs when a blood vessel ruptures and fills a natural cavity of the body.

haematocolpos – menstrual blood held up in the vagina as a result of an imperforate hymen.

haematoma – a collection of blood forming a definite swelling due to injury or an operation; another name for a bruise.

haematuria – passing of blood in the urine.

haemic murmur – an unusual sound heard over the heart or large blood vessels in patients with severe anaemia.

haemochromatosis – a progressive disease characterised by abnormal deposits of iron in many organs of the body. The disease gives rise to cirrhosis of the liver, an enlarged spleen, pigmentation of the skin and diabetes mellitus; sometimes known as bronzed diabetes.

THE FATHER OF MEDICINE?

It was Hippocrates (460-370 BC) – born on the island of Cos and, as a Greek physician, recognised as the Father of Medicine.

He played an important part in laying the foundation of scientific medicine, separating it from philosophical speculation and superstition.

Although the Hippocratic Oath represented his ethical position, it cannot be attributed to him with true confidence.

He travelled widely and taught at the medical school on Cos. When teaching his students he charged a fee.

His idea on the origin of disease was superseded by the germ theory in the 18th and 19th centuries.

haemoglobinopathies – diseases in which there are abnormalities of haemoglobin, either due to defective synthesis or an abnormal form of haemoglobin.

haemoglobinuria – the presence of blood pigment in the urine due to the destruction of red blood corpuscles; present in blackwater fever.

haemolysis – the breaking up of red blood cells, which can be due to the action of poisonous substances such as chemicals, incompatible blood transfusions and snake venom. It can also be due to congenital or acquired conditions leading to haemolytic jaundice and anaemia.

haemolytic disease of the new born – haemolysis or breakdown of the red blood cells due to rhesus incompatibility. In a rhesus negative mother with a rhesus positive foetus, the mother develops antibodies which are passed on to the foetus. This causes the foetal blood cells to break down giving rise to haemolytic anaemia and jaundice in the newborn. (also known as erythroblastosis foetalis).

haemophilia – an hereditary disease occurring predominately in males but carried by the female, which gives rise to a tendency to uncontrollable haemorrhage after a quite slight wound. There is a deficiency of the clotting factor (factor VIII) in the blood. Patients with haemophilia are sometimes known as 'bleeders'. The son of Czar Nicholas II of Russia was a haemophiliac.

haemorrhage – the escape of blood from the vessels containing it.

haemoptysis – coughing or spitting up blood from the lower air passages. It can be due to disease in the lungs such as TB or carcinoma.

haemorrhoids – otherwise known as piles. They are dilated varicose veins around the rectal opening. It is a common condition often tolerated for years and it is sometimes temporary as in pregnancy. They can become painful and may need surgery.

'NOT AN EASY RIDE'?

The Duke of Wellington described the Battle of Waterloo as a close run thing.
Blücher's Prussian troops arrived on the scene at 6 pm as Wellington's army was getting tired and under pressure.
Uncharacteristically, Napoleon had not started his attack until midday allowing the battleground to dry, whereas it was his normal practice to take the field early in the morning.
One of the reasons for this is believed to be that he woke up suffering from an acute attack of haemorrhoids, which made it too painful for the French Emperor to mount his horse and the time it took for the pain to ease was responsible for the late start. Is it possible that a severe case of haemorrhoids (piles) helped the Iron Duke to win the battle?

haemothorax – an effusion of blood into the chest cavity.

hairy tongue – a rare condition where intertwining hairlike filaments form black or brown patches on the tongue. It may occur after the use of antibiotics, but is harmless and usually goes away by itself.

hallux rigidus – stiffness of the joint between the big toe and the foot.

hallux valgus – outward displacement of the great toe. It is caused by the pressure of inappropriate footwear.

halo – a coloured circle round a bright light in some eye conditions. If it is accompanied by headaches it is likely to be caused by glaucoma.

hallucinations – a sensory perception in the absence of a sensory stimulus, usually either visual or auditory.

hamartoma – benign tumours, usually in the lung, which contain the normal components of lung tissue.

hammer toe – a deformity characterised by permanent flexion of the middle joint of the toe. If all the toes are affected, it is known as a claw foot. Usually caused by cramping the foot into too small a shoe.

hand, foot and mouth disease – most common in children. The condition manifests itself by the eruption of blisters on the palm of the hands, on the feet, toes and mouth. It is caused by infection with the coxsackie A16 virus.

Hand-Schuller-Christian disease – an insidiously developing disease occurring in the first decade of life, manifesting itself by bulging eyes, excessive thirst with deposits of cholesterol in the bones and under the skin.

hang nail – a splitting of the skin at the end of the finger nail.

Hansen's disease – leprosy.

hard metal disease – occurs in those who work grinding tungsten carbide. It is characterised by a cough, expectoration and shortness of breath due to inhaling the dust. It is a mild disease, which disappears after ceasing to work with the metal.

hare lip – see cleft palate.

> **Hashimoto's disease** – a condition where there is diffuse enlargement of the thyroid gland. The enlargement is firm and is believed to be due to auto-immunity. The gland is infiltrated with lymphocytes and fibrous tissue.
> The condition is most common in middle aged women. There are no toxic signs, being more like myxoedema in its general effects.

hay fever – an allergic condition affecting the mucous membranes of the eyes, nose and air passages. It is due to a hypersensitivity reaction to pollens of grasses, weeds or trees.

headache – very common but causes vary tremendously from, at one extreme, tumours of the brain and meningitis to a sign of tiredness. The mechanism producing headaches is obscure but it could be due to dilation of the blood vessels to the brain as the brain tissue itself is insensitive to pain. Among many causes are anxiety, migraine, refraction errors of the eye (not common as some think), sinusitis, dental sepsis, indigestion, constipation, fever, uraemia, high blood pressure, sunstroke and diseases of the brain.

heart block – occurs when the transmission of impulses from the atria to the ventricles is interfered with.

heartburn – a burning sensation in the region of the heart and up the back of the throat due to excessive acidity of the gastrointestinal tract with regurgitation. It is relieved by antacids.

heat cramps – painful cramp in the muscles of workers who labour in hot conditions; the result of a loss of salt in the sweat.

heat spots – small inflamed and congested areas on the skin of the face, neck and chest or other parts of the body in warm weather.

heatstroke – a serious reaction to exposure to extreme heat. The heat centres in the brain become paralysed; the victim's extremely high temperature must be reduced immediately with ice packs or cold water.

hebephrenia – a form of schizophrenia coming on in youth with depression and gradual failure of the mental faculties accompanied by self-centred delusions.

Heberden's nodes – little hard nobs which appear at the side of the last phalanges in those suffering from osteoarthrosis (osteoarthritis).

hebetude – mental dullness especially of the temporary variety arising during a fever.

hectic – a type of fever occurring in severe forms of TB or septic poisoning, rising high during the day and falling at night with profuse sweating.

hemeralopia – another name for day blindness.

hemianaesthesia – loss of sense of being touched down the side of the body.

hemianopia – the loss of half the usual area of vision.

hemiatrophy – atrophy of one side or part of the side of the body.

hemiballismus – involuntary choreiform movements but of greater amplitude along with movements of the face. They occur as a result of the vascular damage to the mid-brain.

hemicrania – headaches limited to one side of the head.

hemimelia – defects in the distal parts of the extremities such as the absence of the forearm or hands. A congenital condition e.g. the result of thalidomide administration during pregnancy.

hemiplegia – paralysis limited to one side of the body usually due to a stroke.

Henoch–Schönlein purpura – an allergic form of haemorrhage into the skin, starting with pain in the abdomen and joints. The condition is associated with streptococcal infection, rheumatic fever and food allergy. Recovery is usually spontaneous unless the kidneys are affected.

hepatitis – inflammation of the liver usually due to a virus. If it is non–viral it can be due to an amoeba, alcohol, toxins and syphilis.

hepatolenticular degeneration – see Wilson's disease.

hermaphrodite – an individual in whom both ovarian and testicular tissue are present.

hernia – another name for a rupture. It results in the protrusion of an organ or part of an organ through the cavity which contains it.

herpangina – a short febrile illness with vesicles or 'punched out' ulcers developing in parts of the mouth. The condition is caused by the group A coxsackie virus.

herpes simplex – cold sore or fever blister due to a viral infection.

herpes zoster – another name for shingles.

hiatus hernia – displacement of a portion of the stomach through the opening of the diaphragm through which the oesophagus passes.

> **hiccup** – the spasmodic indrawing of air into the lungs ending with a 'click' due to the sudden closure of the vocal chords. It is caused by the irritation of the nerves which supply the diaphragm.

hip dislocation (congenital) – spontaneous dislocation of the hip joint before or shortly after birth.

hippus – a tremor of the iris giving rise to alternating contraction and dilatation of the pupil. It is often a sign of hysteria.

Hirschsprung's disease – otherwise known as congenital megacolon. It is characterised by great hypertrophy and dilatation of the colon in infants and children.

hirsutism – the growth of hair, of the male type and distribution, in women. It is either due to the excessive production of androgens or the undue sensitivity of hair follicles to normal levels of circulating androgens in females.

histoplasmosis – a systemic infection due to the inhalation of dust containing the spores of the fungus Histoplasma capsulati; most common in the U.S.A.

hives – a popular name for an eruption of the nature of nettle rash.

Hodgkin's disease – a malignant condition affecting the lymph nodes all over the body; otherwise known as lymphadenoma.

homocystinuria – a congenital disease whereby the individual lacks the ability to metabolise or utilize one of the essential amino acids (methionine) properly. It gives rise to abnormalities of the lens of the eye, mental retardation, fair hair and high cheek colour.

honking – a persistent cough of emotional origin occurring in emotionally disturbed children. The noise has been likened to the call of the Canada goose!

hookworm – a disease due to a small worm which enters the body through the skin or by drinking infected water. The parasites pass to the intestines where they "hook" themselves and suck blood, leading to severe anaemia.

hordoleum – an old term for a stye.

Horner's syndrome – a condition which manifests itself by a constricted pupil, a drooping upper eye lid, and an apparent sunken eye, caused by paralysis of the sympathetic nerve in the neck. It is usually caused by pressure on the sympathetic nerve by secondary spread from cancer of the lung to a lymph gland in the neck.

horripilation – gooseflesh. It is caused by the contraction of small muscles in the skin making the hairs erect.

horseshoe kidney – kidneys linked at their lower ends by a band of tissue instead of being separate, resembling a horseshoe. It can sometimes give rise to complications such as hydronephrosis, pyelonephritis and renal stones.

humidifier fever – a form of alveolitis caused by the contamination of water used to humidify or moisten air in air conditioning systems.

Huntingdon's chorea – an hereditary disease characterised by involuntary movements and dementia. Each child of a parent with the disease stands a 50:50 chance of developing it. It usually comes on between the ages of 35 and 45 but some 10% start under 20 years of age. It is estimated that there are some 6000 cases in Britain. There is no effective treatment.

Hurler's syndrome – see gargoylism.

Hutchinson's teeth – widely spaced, narrow edged upper central incisors with notches at the biting edge; usually a sign of congenital syphilis.

hyaline membrane disease – a condition found in premature infants with difficulty in breathing occurring a few hours after birth. The affected infant cannot get enough oxygen because the ducts leading to the tiny air sacs in the lungs are lined with a thin membrane, probably derived from the baby's own secretions. It is also known as 'respiratory distress syndrome'; the mortality rate is over 50%.

hydatid disease – infestation with animal tapeworms which produce clusters of fluid filled cysts in the lungs and other organs.

hydatidiform mole – rare complication of early pregnancy due to degeneration of membranes which normally become part of the placenta. There is a proliferation of the epithelium of the outer two membranes. Immediate evacuation of the uterus is necessary. The other name for the condition is 'vesicular mole'.

hydradenitis suppurativa – a chronic inflammatory disease of the apocose sweat glands (armpits, around anus and external genitals). More common in women, but occurs in the men who drive lorries and taxis; painful tender lumps are present under the skin.

hydraemia – condition in which the blood contains an excess of water.

hydramnios – excess fluid in the amniotic cavity in pregnancy.

hydrocephalus – water on the brain; abnormal amounts of cerebrospinal fluid in the brain cavity exert pressure on the brain substance which becomes damaged.

hydrocoele – a swelling of the scrotum from the accumulation of fluid in the sac of the membrane that covers the testicles.

hydronephrosis – a chronic disease of the kidney which becomes distended with fluid, usually due to an obstruction to the outflow of urine; most commonly the result of a stone or stricture within the kidney, ureter or bladder.

hydrophobia – another name for rabies.

hydrops foetalis – extreme result of haemolytic disease of the newborn; oedema occurs in the foetus due to accumulation of excess fluid in the pericardial, pleural and peritoneal cavities.

hydrothrax – a collection of fluid in the thoracic cavity.

hyperacusis – an abnormally acute sense of hearing.

hyperaemia – the presence of an excessive amount of blood in the vessels supplying an organ or a part of the body.

hyperaesthesia – oversensitivity of a part; most common in some diseases of the central nervous system.

> **hyperalgesia** – excessive sensitiveness to pain.

hypercalciuria – an abnormally large amount of calcium in the urine.

hypercapnia – an abnormally large amount of carbon dioxide in the blood or lungs.

hyperchlorhydria – excess production of hydrochloric acid in the gastric juice.

hypercholesteraemia – an excessive amount of cholesterol in the bloodstream.

hyperemesis – excessive vomiting.

hyperemesis gravidorum – a severe form of vomiting in pregnancy, which is greater than in morning sickness; it may require admission to hospital.

hyperglycaemia – an excessive amount of sugar in the blood; it is found in untreated diabetes mellitus.

hyperhidrosis – an excessive amount of sweating.

hyperlipidaemia – an excessive amount of fats found in the blood, which can either be due to cholesterol (in atheroma or coronary heart disease) or triglycerides (in pancreatitis).

hypermetropia – another name for longsightedness.

hypernephroma – a malignant tumour in the kidney usually occurring in those over the age of 40.

hyperpiesis – another name for high blood pressure.

hyperplasia – an abnormal increase in the number of cells in an organ or tissue, with a consequent enlargement of the part affected.

hyperpyrexia – an excessively high temperature.

hypersensitivity – an abnormal immunological response in certain individuals; an allergic reaction.

hypertelorism – a rare congenital deformity of the head and face (known as totem pole head).

hypertension – abnormally high arterial blood pressure.

hyperthermia – abnormally high temperature (hyperpyrexia).

hyperthyroidism – an excess activity of the thyroid gland as in Graves' disease.

hypertrophy – an increase in size of an organ without an increase in the number of cells; usually due to overactivity.

> **hyperventilation** – another name for overbreathing, with a consequent lowering of carbon dioxide in the blood, which can lead to loss of consciousness.

hypocalcaemia – low blood calcium.

hypochlorhydria – a low level of hydrochloric acid in the gastric juice.

hypochondriasis – a chronic mental condition in which the affected person is continually occupied with the delusion that he or she is ill.

hypoglycaemia – a deficiency of the sugar in the blood; may be due to starvation or occur after receiving insulin.

hypogonadism – a condition caused by the deficiency of hormones produced by the gonads.

hypomania – a slight degree of mania.

hypopiesis – an abnormally low blood pressure.

hypoplasia – incomplete or arrested development of an organ or part.

hypopon – a collection of pus in the antechamber of the eye.

hypospadias – a congenital malformation in which the urethra fails to fuse completely, leaving an open channel on the underside of the penis.

hypostasis – the accumulation of blood or fluid in a part of the body due to poor circulation; when it occurs in the lungs hypostatic pneumonia can develop which can be a terminal condition, particularly in elderly bedridden patients.

> **hypotension** – abnormally low blood pressure.

hypothermia – excessively low temperature; this condition is a particular problem with elderly people living on their own in winter.

hypothyroidism – defective action of the thyroid gland (see myxoedema).

> **hysteria** – a nervous condition characterised by susceptibility to suggestion, emotional instability, amnesia and other mental abnormality.

iatrogenic disease – a disease induced, unintentionally, by the words or actions of the physician; most often due to the actions of drugs administered to treat the patient's condition.

ichthyosis – a skin disease in which the surface is very rough and dry with the appearance of fish scales; the condition is hereditary.

icterus – another name for jaundice.

icterus gravis neonatorum – another name for haemolytic disease of the newborn.

ictus – another name for a stroke.

idioglossus – continual utterance of meaningless sounds.

idiosyncrasy – a peculiar personal capacity to react abnormally to drugs, foods or treatments; a constitutional defect in the individual.

ileitis – inflammation of the ileum; it gives rise to colicky abdominal pain, irregular bowel movements, loss of weight and sometimes slight loss of blood. Can be due to Crohn's disease.

ileostomy – an operation in which an artificial opening is made into the ileum; it is usually carried out in people with chronic large bowel disease.

ileus – paralysis of the bowel muscle.

illusion – an erroneous concept or belief or an erroneous perception of reality; a sign in a number of mental conditions. An example is the mistaken belief that an object is someone known to the individual. During one of his periods of insanity King George III shook hands with an oak tree in the mistaken belief that it was Frederick the Great, Emperor of Prussia!

imbecility – severe subnormality.

immersion foot – a condition which develops as a result of prolonged immersion of the feet in cold water; it causes constriction of the small arteries giving rise to coldness, blueness or even gangrene of the affected foot (as in trench foot).

impaction – applied to a condition in which two ends are firmly lodged together as in a fracture; also a term applied to a condition where there is abnormal placement in an alveolus preventing normal eruption as in impacted wisdom teeth.

imperstix – infantilism or imperfect sexual development.

impetigo – an infectious skin disease characterised by pustules that burst and form thick yellow crusts. The condition is caused by the bacterium Staphylococcus aureus and the infection most often appears on the face. In young children it is known as pemphigus neonatorum and requires urgent treatment.

impotence – inability to perform the sexual act.

incompetence – a condition applied to the valves of the heart either due to disease or due to relative enlargement of the heart chambers so that the valves are unable to function properly.

ANAESTHETICS

Most of the operations referred to in this book would not have been possible without the discovery of anaesthetics.

In the past there were disputes as to who was the first to administer general anaesthesia, but it is now accepted that the first properly recorded operation to be carried out thus was by James C. Warren, an American surgeon. The anaesthetic, ether, was administered by a former dentist William Thomas Green Morton, in 1846, to Warren's patient Gilbert Abbot from whom a tumour of the neck was to be removed.

The operation was carried out in Warren's operating theatre in Boston in front of a highly sceptical audience of medical students.

When Warren made his incision and the patient neither moved nor cried out, the surgeon said to his assistants and the students, "Gentlemen, this is no humbug"!

incontinence – the inability to retain urine or faeces.

incoordination – the inability to exercise normal voluntary control of relatively complex muscular movements.

indigestion – either inadequate or excess secretion of the gastric digestive juice. It presents as pain in the heart region or shooting up to the right shoulder soon after eating food. Also called dyspepsia.

infantile paralysis – old term for poliomyelitis.

infantilism – imperfect sexual development at puberty; condition may or may not be associated with smallness of stature; normally due to a lack or shortage of hormones secreted by the pituitary or adrenal glands.

infarction – an area of dead tissue due to complete blockage of its blood supply.

infection – the process by which disease is communicated from one person to others. It can be caused by different types of organism e.g. bacteria, viruses and others.

infectious mononucleosis – another name for glandular fever.

infertility – the inability to produce children.

infestation – the presence of animal parasites in the intestine or other organs.

inflammation – the reaction of tissue to injury. The injury may be due to trauma or infection.

influenza – an acute infection due to a virus usually occurring in epidemics.

inhibition – the arrest or restraint of some process by the influence of the nervous system.

insomnia – the inability to sleep.

intermittent claudication – pain in the leg or legs after walking a certain distance, which is relieved by resting; it may be due to arteriosclerosis or other arterial disease (see Buerger's disease).

intertrigo – redness, abrasion and maceration of opposing skin surfaces which rub together.

intoxication – term applied to states of poisoning.

introspection – observation of one's thoughts or feelings.

intussusception – a form of obstruction of the intestine where one part enters another part immediately adjacent to it; most common in infants.

involution – the process of change when the uterus returns to its normal state after childbirth.

iodism – condition caused by the overdose of iodine or iodine compounds.

iridectomy – a hole made in the iris to treat glaucoma.

irritable bowel syndrome – the overreaction of the colon to emotions or other stimuli, without obvious organic cause. Symptoms include pain in the lower abdomen, distension and abdominal aching.

ischaemia – local deficiency of blood supply due to spasm or obstruction of an artery.

ischaemic heart disease – see coronary thrombosis.

ischio-rectal abscess – an abscess occurring in the space between the rectum and the ischial bone of the pelvis.

ischuria – insufficiency in amount of urine either due to the suppression of excretion or the reduction of the kidney.

itch – the popular name for scabies.

itching – an unpleasant condition of the skin surface (pruritis).

Jacksonian epilepsy – convulsions starting in a single muscle or a group of muscles. Consciousness is usually maintained. It may proceed to grand mal (qv). The condition may be due to a localised lesion in the brain such as a tumour.

Japanese encephalitis – a virus infection which occurs in eastern Asia; transmitted by the bite of a mosquito.

jail fever – another name for typhus fever.

jaundice – a yellow discolouration of the skin due to the deposition of bile pigments in the deeper layers. The underlying abnormality may be in the liver itself, the bile passages outside the liver or in the blood. If the red cells of the blood break down the condition is known as haemolytic jaundice. The first sign may be a yellowish tinge in the whites of the eyes.

joint mice – a popular name for loose bodies in a joint, particularly the knee.

K

kala-azar – another name for visceral Leishmaniasis, an infection transmitted by the bite of sand-flies occurring in the Mediterranean, tropical and oriental regions. It is characterised by fever, anaemia, enlarged spleen and emaciation. The condition has a high mortality rate if left untreated.

> **Kaposi's sarcoma** – localised red or purple, flat or raised lesion occurring anywhere on the body like a mini-bruise. A malignant complication of AIDS. 25% of AIDS sufferers present with this.

kaolinosis – a form of pneumoconiosis caused by inhaling clay dust.

Kawasaki disease – a disease of childhood usually occurring between 6 months and 2 years and is characterised by a high fever, conjunctivitis, skin rash and swollen neck glands. The acute stage clears spontaneously, but complications can include arteritis and coronary artery aneurisms. The condition was first described in Japan but it now has spread to Europe.

keloid – the overgrowth of fibrous tissue usually on the site of an old scar of a previous injury or operation.

keratitis – inflammation of the cornea of the eye. Viral keratitis is due to the herpes simplex virus.

keratoconjunctivitis – acute inflammation of the cornea and conjunctiva which often occurs in epidemics. It is caused by a specific virus.

keratomalacia – a softening of the cornea due to severe vitamin A deficiency.

keratosis – a disease of the skin characterised by the overgrowth of the horny layer. It can give rise to a wart or a callus; but it may be induced by exposure to sunlight.

kerion – a suppurating form of ringworm.

kernicterus – staining of the basal nuclei of the brain with bile, which can be a severe complication of haemolytic disease of the newborn.

Kernig's sign – a sign of meningeal irritation when bending the thigh with the knee straight causes pain in the back of the neck.

ketosis – occurs when more fat is eaten than the body can burn completely. The unburned fats produce chemicals called ketone bodies, which give rise to a form of acidosis to which some diabetics are susceptible.

Kimmelsteil-Wilson disease – a specific form of kidney disease associated with long standing diabetes.

king's evil – another name for scrofula, a defective nutritional disease of the tissues rendering the sufferer susceptible to tuberculosis. It was thought to be curable by the touch of the royal hand.

kleptomania – an irresistible compulsion to steal things without necessarily needing them and regardless of their value.

> **Klinefelter's syndrome** – a condition originally described as gynaecomastia, testicular atrophy and infertility with intelligence unimpaired. Cases have since been described with associated mental defects. A person with Klinefelter's syndrome has an extra X chromosome so the male has XXY instead of XY in his chromosomal make up.

knock-knees – otherwise known as genu valgum. A condition whereby when the legs are straightened they diverge from one another and as a result when walking the knees knock together; in young children it corrects itself spontaneously.

Köhler's disease – osteochondritis of the navicular bone of the hand; the condition resolves spontaneously, but a return to playing sports and games should be gradual.

koilonychia – a term applied when the nails are hollowed out and depressed like a spoon; associated with chronic iron deficiency.

Koplik's spots – small bluish white spots appearing on the mucous membranes in the mouth. They present shortly before the measles rash appears.

Korsakow's syndrome (or psychosis) – a mental disturbance occurring in chronic alcoholism and other toxic states such as uraemia, lead poisoning and syphilis. Manifestations of the condition include loss of memory for recent events, falsification of memory, talkativeness and delusions with regards to time and place although clear in other matters, such as the description of imaginary journeys and what the person has seen in the distant places.

kraurosis – a progressive drying of the skin due to atrophy of the glands and associated with shrivelling and itching; it occurs in the vulva of elderly women.

Kummel's disease – a condition resulting from an undiagnosed crush fracture of the vertebra due to injury

kuru – a slowly progressive disease caused by degeneration in the central nervous system, particularly the cerebellum. It occurs in the Fore people of the east highlands of New Guinea. It is caused by a slow virus infection acquired from eating the organs, especially the brains, of diseased relations (eaten out of respect!). It originally occurred in women and children who practised this rite. This has now been given up but kuru still occurs in some women as it has an incubation period of 20 years.

kwashiorkor – one of the most important causes of ill health and death among children in the tropics. The disease is the result of a diet deficient in protein and so called essential fatty acids, where the infants weaned from the breast are unable to cope with an adult diet.

kyphosis – forward curvature of the spine.

![L]

lactose intolerance – a condition due to the lack of the enzyme lactase; the body thus being unable to digest lactose, the sugar in milk; more common in coloured races.

Laennec's cirrhosis – another name for portal cirrhosis, the most common form of cirrhosis of the liver.

lagophthalmos – a condition in which the eye cannot be completely closed.

laparotomy – a term applied to any operation in which the abdomen is opened.

laryngismus stridulus – a form of spasmodic croup occurring in children at night without prodromal symptoms. Children affected grow out of it.

laryngitis – inflammation of the mucous membrane of the larynx; it can be acute or chronic and is usually caused by a virus infection, but it can be due to a bacterial infection or due to voice abuse (traumatic).

laryngo-tracheo-bronchitis – acute infection of the respiratory tract in infants and young children; it is usually caused by a virus but it may be due to an infection by the bacteria Haemophilus influenzae. It presents as a croupy cough and stridulous breathing. The child requires immediate medical attention.

Lassa fever – a condition first reported in Lassa, Nigeria; the disease is caused by an arenavirus which can be transmitted by rodents or infected persons. The condition presents as fever, headaches, lethargy, rash (due to bleeding under the skin and mucous membranes), muscular pain and sore throat; there is a high mortality rate particularly in pregnancy.

lathyrism – a disease characterised by pain and paralysis of the legs caused by eating a variety of chick-pea.

> **Laurence-Moon-Biedl syndrome** – a rare genetic disorder of the pituitary gland producing obesity, mental retardation, degeneration of the retina, webbed fingers or toes, underdevelopment of the genitals and six fingers on each hand.

lead poisoning – poisoning due to the absorption of lead or its salts into the body. The condition may be acute or chronic due to accumulation of the metal over a long period of time. The signs of chronic lead poisoning are abdominal pain, constipation, muscle weakness, pallor, drowsiness, mental confusion and a blue line in the gums.

Leber's disease – an hereditary disease in which blindness comes on at about the age of twenty.

> **legionnaire's disease** – a form of pneumonia due to the organism Legionella pneumophilia. The organisms thrive in static water tanks which provide favourable conditions for multiplication. They also thrive in water aerosols. The condition is characterised by breathlessness, fever, chest pain and dry cough.

The term 'Legionnaire's Disease' has no connection with the French Foreign Legion. It is derived from a 1976 state convention of the American Legion, a war veteran's organisation at a Philadelphia hotel, where 182 Legionnaires contracted the disease, 29 of them fatally. Medical detective work by the U.S. centre for disease control in Atlanta, Georgia, pieced together clues and laboratory work, It discovered that the organism had many unique properties and was unlike any other known bacterium previously encountered. Later studies of stored samples revealed that a number of mysterious outbreaks at widely separated places were episodes of Legionnaire's disease.

leiomyoma – a tumour made up of unstriped or involuntary muscle.

Leishmaniasis – a parasitic disease transmitted by certain sandflies. The variety caused by the protozoan organism Leishmania donovani is also known as Dum-Dum fever.

lentigo – another name for freckles.

leprosy – a chronic disease affecting particularly the skin, mucous membranes and nerves, caused by the organism Mycobacterium leprosi; it is a disease of low infectivity, but it can give rise to deformities and mutilations. It is also known as Hansen's disease.

leptomeningitis – inflammation of the inner and more delicate membranes of the brain and spinal cord.

leptospirosis – an infectious disease caused by the spirochaete Leptospira icterohaemorrhagica, caninola and hebiornalis. The former gives rise to Weil's disease which is transmitted by rat's urine and can occur in sewage workers. It is characterised by fever, jaundice, enlarged liver and bleeding from the mucous membranes.

leucocytosis – an abnormal increase in the numbers of white cells in the blood. It occurs most commonly as a defence against infection and inflammation. There is a slight increase in pregnancy, during the menstrual cycle and during exercise.

leucodermia – areas of the skin become white as a result of skin disease.

> **leucopenia** – a diminished number of white blood cells; it may result from allergies, drug reactions, irradiation, some infections and anaemias.

leucoplakia – a chronic condition whereby white leathery patches appear on the tongue, the mucous membranes of the mouth and on the vulva. Irritation is believed to be a factor causing the condition and lesions in the mouth tend to improve if the sufferer stops smoking.

leucorrhoea – a whitish discharge from the vagina. The condition often occurs during ovulation, but it may be due to a yeast or protozoal infection.

leukaemia – a malignant condition of the blood forming organs. It is characterised by a gross overproduction of white blood cells.

lichen – a term applied to a group of chronic skin diseases characterised by thickening and hardness of the skin with the formation of papules.

lichen planus – an itching eruption of unknown cause where dull purplish spots appear on thin skinned areas of the body.

lick eczema – an irritating eruption around the mouth of children who persistently lick their lips or suck their thumb.

lienteric diarrhoea – a mild form of diarrhoea where the bowels move soon after meals.

lightning injuries – injuries caused by being struck by lightning.

lipidystrophy – a congenital maldistribution of fat tissue where subcutaneous fat is absent from parts of the body and hypertrophied in the remainder. An acquired form occurs at the site of insulin injections.

lipoma – a benign tumour composed mainly of fat found in almost any part of the body but principally in fibrous tissue beneath the skin.

lippitudo – a chronic condition manifested by inflammation at the margins of the eyelids.

listeriosis – an infectious disease of animals sometimes transmitted to man affecting the central nervous system by causing meningitis and encephalitis. It sometimes occurs in the newborn, transmitted from their mother through the placenta. The organism concerned is Listeria monocytogenes.

lithiasis – a general term given to the formation of calculi.

lithopaedion – a condition whereby a foetus having died in the mother's body becomes calcified.

Little's disease – a form of cerebral palsy, affecting both sides of the body, in children.

live-flesh – a popular term applied to fine muscular tremors or twitching seen especially in the eyelids and muscles of the hands. Usually due to tiredness or to overuse of the particular muscles, but if it is persistent it may be a sign of a serious nervous disease.

liver fluke – a disease acquired by ingesting food or water contaminated with the cysts of the sheep liver fluke, a type of flatworm.

liver spot – brownish marks appearing on the skin frequently seen in pregnancy. It can sometimes be due to the parasite Tinea versicola in the surface area of the epithelium.

loasis – a disease caused by the filarial worm Loa Loa, a worm shorter than W.bancrofti which enters the bloodstream during the day. It is transmitted by the mango fly, Chrysops dimidiata.
The condition occurs in Central Africa and causes lumps anywhere in the body as the worm migrates.
It is usually found in the eye under the conjunctiva.

lockjaw – a prominent symptom of, and another name for, tetanus.

locomotor ataxia – another name for tabes dorsalis, a disease affecting the central nervous system occurring in the tertiary stage of syphilis.

logorrhoea – a technical term for garrulousness, a feature which may be exaggerated in certain states of mental instability.

lordosis – an unnatural forward curvature of the spine.

lues – a Latin word for serious infectious diseases, especially applied to syphilis.

lumbago – a general term for pain in the muscles of the lumbar region, usually of rheumatic origin.

lunatic – a general term applied to people with a disordered mind, who were thought to be influenced by the moon.

lupus erythematosus – a chronic inflammatory disease affecting the skin and internal organs and characterised by a scaly red rash on the face; it is believed to be due to auto-immunity.

lupus vulgaris – a form of tuberculosis of the skin characterised by ulcerating nodular facial lesions especially around the nose and ears.

luxation – another name for dislocation.

lycanthropy – a delusion by an insane person who believes that he or she is a wolf.

lymphadenitis – inflammation of the lymph glands.

lymphadenoma – another name for Hodgkin's disease.

lymphangiectasis – abnormal dilation of the lymph vessels like that which occurs in filariasis.

lymphoedema – swelling of a part of an organ due to obstruction of the lymph vessels as in elephantiasis.

lymphogranuloma inguinale – a venereal disease of viral origin characterised by an enlargement of the lymph glands in the groin; otherwise known as lymphogranuloma venereum.

lymphoma – any of various malignant tumours of the lymph nodes or lymphoid tissue.

lymphosarcoma – a malignant growth of the lymphoid elements of the body often characterised by general enlargement of the lymph glands, the liver or spleen.

lysis – a gradual ending of a fever as opposed to 'crisis' which is a sudden ending. Lysis is also the term given to the dissolution of a blood clot or the loosening of adhesions.

> **lysol poisoning** – a very severe form of poisoning due to the ingestion of lysol; it gives rise to unconsciousness, stupor and death within 24 hours or goes on to cause septic pneumonia. For treatment tepid water and salt should be given to dilute the lysol before causing vomiting.

lyssa – another term for rabies or hydrophobia.

maceration – a softening and deterioration of tissue in constant and confined contact with liquids.

macrofisa – a disease of the macula in the eye where objects appear larger than normal.

macroglossia – an abnormally large tongue.

macule – a flat discoloured spot on the surface of the skin (the rash of measles is macular).

Madura foot – a chronic fungus infection of the foot occurring in tropical regions; the swollen foot becomes filled with cyst like areas connected by sinuses, from which the fungus containing pus drains. In time the disease destroys the tissue and amputation may be necessary.

maidism – another name for pellagra.

malabsorption syndrome – a descriptive term for a number of disorders which result from defective absorption of essential foodstuffs by the small intestine. The term covers conditions such as coeliac disease, sprue and idiopathic steatorrhoea and involves foodstuffs such as fats, vitamins and mineral salts.

malacia – a term applied to the softening of a part or of tissue in disease.

malaise – a vague feeling of feverishness, listlessness, languor and other symptoms which may precede the onset of a serious acute disease.

> **malaria** – a disease caused by one of the malarial parasites (such as Plasmodium vivax, P.falciparum or P.malariae) in the blood. The parasites are transmitted by the female anopheles mosquito. The disease is characterised by cycles of chills, fever and sweating. Treatment can be either preventative or curative.

malignant fever – a rare but dangerous complication of general anaesthesia. It is characterised by a sudden rise in temperature (hyperthermia) during anaesthesia after a few minutes or several hours. It is often associated with familial abnormalities in the muscle.

> Sir Ronald Ross (1822-1884) proved that the tropical illness malaria is caused by a germ carried by the anopheles mosquito.
>
> Before that, it was thought to be caused by bad air or water.

malingering – feigning illness.

mallet finger – a sudden forced flexion of the terminal joint of a finger resulting in rupture of the tendon. The sufferer is then unable to extend the terminal part of the finger; the middle and ring fingers are most commonly involved.

mallet toe – similar to mallet finger but usually due to a muscular imbalance which may be caused by a congenital absence of the extensor muscle.

Malta fever – another name for brucellosis.

manic-depressive insanity – a form of madness where there are alternate attacks of mania and depression (cyclothymia).

marasmus – a progressive wasting and emaciation especially in young infants. There may be no ascertainable cause or it may be due to defective feeding.

Marburg disease – a fatal virus disease which is transmitted to humans from the vervet or green monkey by contact with infected tissue. A number of cases have been reported in Africa.The disease presents with a rising temperature, diarrhoea and vomiting. A rash and internal bleeding appear after nearly a week. The disease is named after the West German city where a laboratory technician contracted it in 1967.

> **march fracture** – a fracture of the second (or rarely the third) metatarsal bone of the foot without obvious cause. It can develop while walking.

march haemoglobinuria – a complication of walking or running over long distances where damage is caused to the blood vessels in the soles of the feet. The haemoglobin is released into the blood stream and voided in the urine. The condition can be minimised by wearing shoes with more resistant soles.

Marfan's syndrome – another name for arachnodactyly.

Marie-Strumpell disease – another name for ankylosing spondylitis.

marsh fever – another name for malaria.

mastalgia – another name for pain in the breast.

mastitis – inflammation of the breasts due to bacterial or other causes. The most common disease of the female breast is chronic mastitis, where the breast contains nodules and small cysts, which are frequently painful.

mastoiditis – inflammation of the mastoid bone just behind the ear, the result of infection spreading from either acute or chronic middle ear infection.

mat burn – a burn or abrasion occurring in a wrestler when the skin over the bony prominences rub over the canvas mat; the condition can become infected.

mattoid – a person, though passing as sane, is eccentric or mentally unbalanced in some way.

M.E. – see myeloencephalopathy.

measles – acute infectious disease occurring in children. Measles (or morbilli) is caused by a virus and, although most children recover from an attack without serious side effects, it can give rise to encephalitis and mental retardation or chronic lung damage. This makes it necessary to protect children from the disease by vaccination.

> American physician Henry Koplik in 1896 identified the so called Koplik spots which appear in the mouth of measles patients only. Their presence, apart from being a diagnostic sign of measles, provided a basis for differential diagnosis between measles and rubella.

Meckel's diverticulum – a blind opening two to five inches long coming from the small intestine. It normally is obliterated during foetal development but it can persist in some people as a vestigeal remnant. If it becomes inflamed it can cause symptoms resembling appendicitis.

megalomania – a mental condition where the individual has delusions of grandeur and an insane belief in the person's own extreme greatness, goodness or power.

megrim – another name for migraine.

melaena – the passing of dark stools due to bleeding in the higher parts of the bowel or stomach. The dark or black colour is due to the blood having undergone chemical changes on the way down to the bowel.

melancholia – a mental condition characterised by a feeling of dejection and usually by withdrawal. It is often a phase of manic-depressive psychosis.

melanoma – a tumour arising from cells which produce the pigment melanin. A malignant melanoma is a highly malignant form arising from the pigmented cells of moles.

melorheostosis – an abnormal condition of bones with abnormal hardening and denseness extending in a linear direction through one of the long bones of the limb causing deformity and limitation of movement.

Menière's disease – a condition first described in 1861 by Prosper Menière. It manifests itself by tinnitus, deafness and intermittent attacks of vertigo. The disease usually comes on in middle age, occurring in men slightly more than women. There may be gaps of a few weeks to months between attacks and is due to an excessive amount of fluid in the labyrinth of the inner ear.

meningism – a condition found in feverish states where there are symptoms resembling meningitis.

meningitis – an inflammation affecting the membranes of the brain (cerebral) or the spinal cord (spinal). The condition is accompanied by temperature, headaches, vomiting, photophobia and stiffness or rigidity of the neck. It can be caused by a virus infection or a variety of different bacterial organisms e.g. tuberculosis, syphilis, pneumococcus, meningococcus, Haemophilus influenzae and others.

meningocoele – a protrusion of the meninges through a defect in the spine.

meningoencephalitis – an inflammation affecting the meninges and the underlying brain.

meningomyelocoele – protrusion of meninges through a defect in the spine.

menopause – a cessation of menstruation at the end of reproductive life.

menorrhagia – excessive bleeding at the time of a period.

meralgia paraesthetica – pain and paraesthesia occurring on the front or outer aspect of the thigh. It is more common in men than women, in those of middle age, over weight and out of condition. The condition is due to compression of the lateral cutaneous nerve of the thigh.

mercury poisoning – may be acute, due to swallowing a solution containing mercury salts, or chronic, due to long term exposure to mercury or its salts. The manifestations of acute poisoning are pain in the mouth and stomach, then diarrhoea and vomiting and a metallic taste in the mouth. Among the signs and symptoms of chronic poisoning are an increased discharge of saliva into the mouth, bad breath, tender and spongy gums with bleeding and loose and broken teeth. More general signs include trembling and palsy.

metatarsalgia – pain in the foot affecting the metatarsal bones which can be a manifestation of rheumatoid arthritis. Morton's metatarsalgia is associated with damage to the nerve to the 2nd toe crest due to compression by tight shoes.

meteorism – a distension of the abdomen by gas produced in the intestine.

methaemoglobinaemia – the presence in the blood of methaemoglobin with the skin and the lips tinged blue accompanied by breathlessness, headache fatigue and sickness. The condition is either hereditary or toxic due to certain drugs including acetinalide, phenacetin, sulphanilamide and benzocaine. It can be caused by excess nitrates in the drinking water.

metritis – inflammation of the womb.

metropathia haemorrhagica – a condition characterised by haemorrhage from the uterus usually associated with small cysts in the ovaries and thickening of the uterine mucous membrane. The condition is due to the unopposed action of excessive amounts of oestrogens produced by the ovaries.

metrorrhagia – bleeding from the womb otherwise than at the normal period time.

microangiopathy – disease of the capillaries.

microcephaly – abnormal smallness of the head.

micropsia – a disease of the macula in which objects seem smaller than normal.

migraine – sometimes known as hemicrania; a condition characterised by intense headaches occurring in women more often than men. The condition usually only affects one side of the head and is often accompanied by nausea. The attacks can be provoked by certain foods, alcohol, prolonged lack of food, irregular meals, anxiety and other factors.

milia – small keratin cysts appearing as white papules on the cheeks or eyelids.

miliaria – a group of disorders of the skin due to disorders of perspiration.

miosis – a condition where there is excessive contraction of the pupil.

mithraditism – immunity against poisoning by the administration of increasing doses of the poison itself.

mitral stenosis – a narrowing of the opening between the left atrium and the left ventricle due to disease of the valve; most frequently caused by rheumatic fever.

mogigraphia – writer's cramp.

mongolism – another name for Down's syndrome.

Mongolian blue spots – irregular shaped areas of bluish black pigmented skin found occasionally on the buttocks, lower limbs or upper arms of newborn infants of African, Chinese or Japanese parents. They are often mistaken for burns.

moniliasis – an infection due to the fungus Candida albicans normally occurring in the mouth or vagina (thrush), lungs, intestine, skin or nails.

monkey pox – a virus small pox like infection occurring in monkeys kept in captivity. There have been a small number of cases reported in humans in the equatorial rainfall areas of Zaire and West and Central Africa.

monomania – a form of insanity where the person has a delusion on one subject.

monoplegia – paralysis of a single limb or part.

Mooren's ulcer – a particular form of peripheral corneal ulceration.

morbilli – another name for measles.

moron – a mentally subnormal person with a mental age between 8–12.

morphoea – a form of circumscribed scleroderma.

motor neuron disease – a disease caused by the degeneration of the anterior horn cells of the grey matter of the spinal chord. The condition can also refer to the degeneration and wasting of the nerve cells in the bulb of the brain from which the cranial nerves originate. The condition gives rise to spastic paralysis and wasting of the muscles.

motion sickness – nausea and vomiting brought on by forms of motion which rotate the head simultaneously in more than one plane e.g. sea sickness, car sickness, train sickness and air sickness.

mountain sickness – a temporary condition brought on by diminished amounts of oxygen in the air at high altitudes.

mouth ulcers – little blisters on the mucous membranes of the mouth and cheeks which break and leave open sores; otherwise known as aphthous ulcers.

mucocoele – an abnormally dilated cavity in the body due to the accumulation of mucus.

mucocutaneous lymph node syndrome – a condition which occurs in Japan, Korea, Hawaii, Greece and the U.S.A in children under 5. It is characterised by fever, rash, enlarged glands of the neck, the rash being bright red on the hands and feet. Sometimes there are complications such as meningitis, jaundice and myocarditis.

mucomembranous colic – a condition characterised by abdominal pain, constipation and the passage of mucus in the stools. The spasms of colic may be due to an allergy and the condition is most common in highly strung neurotic people.

mucous patch – a syphilitic eruption affecting the mucous membranes particularly in the mouth, the throat and on the lips. The condition is very infectious.

mucoviscidosis – another name for cystic fibrosis or fibrocystic disease of the pancreas.

multiple sclerosis – a degenerative disease of the brain and spinal cord in which the sheaths surrounding individual nerve cells of the brain or spinal cord or both are damaged causing disorders of speech, vision and muscle coordination along with partial paralysis.

mumps – a virus infection, acutely infectious, causing swelling of the parotid and other salivary glands. It is otherwise known as epidemic parotitis and complications include meningitis, encephalitis and pancreatitis, as well as orchitis.

murmur – an abnormal sound usually in the thoracic cavity originating from the heart or lungs and detectable by ear or a stethoscope.

muscae volitantes – spots and threads before the eyes, another term for floaters.

muscular dystrophy – a chronic congenital wasting disease in which complete incapacity follows gradual irreversible muscular deterioration. The muscle is replaced by fatty tissue.

mushroom worker's lung – a lung disease due to hypersensitivity to mushrooms.

myaesthenia gravis – a chronic disease characterised by rapid fatigue of certain muscles followed by a prolonged time to recover their function. The muscles most commonly affected are those of the eyes, making it difficult to raise the eyelids, and of the throat. It is believed to be an auto-immune disease affecting the transmission of acetyl choline across the motor end plate. It is sometimes associated with an enlarged thymus gland.

myalgia – pain in a muscle.

myalgic encephalomyelitis – a disease of viral origin occurring in epidemics and characterised by fever, meningism, double vision, urinary retention and sensory changes. It is also known as epidemic neuraesthenia.

mycosis – a disease due to the growth of fungi (e.g. Candida albicans) in the body.

mycosis fungoides – a rare neoplastic condition of the reticulo-endothelial system giving rise to multiple tumours of the skin, usually with a fatal outcome.

mydriasis – a condition where there is prolonged and abnormal dilatation of the pupil as a result of disease or drugs.

myelitis – inflammation of the spinal cord or bone marrow.

myeloencephalopathy (M.E.) – see post-viral fatigue syndrome.

myeloma – a malignant tumour made up of bone marrow cells usually occurring in the bone marrow itself.

myelomalacia – a softening of the spinal cord as a result of injury pressure, arterial disease or inflammation.

myelomatosis – a malignant process involving the bone marrow.

myiasis – infestation of human tissue by fly maggots or a disease caused by them.

myocarditis – inflammation of the muscular wall of the heart.

myoclonus – brief twitching and muscular contractions involving single or many muscles.

myoma – a tumour consisting of muscle fibres, often occurring in the uterus (fibroid).

myopathy – any disease of muscles.

myopia – short–sightedness.

myositis – inflammation of a muscle.

myotonia – a muscle possessed of normal power but contracting very slowly with tonic spasm and muscular rigidity.

myxoedema – a disease caused by underactivity of the thyroid gland (hypothroidism) in adults. The condition is characterised by dry skin, swelling around the lips and nose (puffy face), mental deterioration and a subnormal basal metabolic rate. It can be controlled by the administration of thyroid extracts or thyroxine.

myxoma – a tumour consisting of very imperfect connective tissue with elements of mucous.

N

naevus – a local area of pigmentation or elevation of the skin, often due to a mass of dilated blood vessels; a mole or birthmark. It can be any malformation of the skin present at birth.

nappy rash – eruptions occurring on the buttocks of infants due to infrequent changes of soiled nappies or inadequate laundering; more common in bottle fed babies. The rash is usually the result of ammonia burns from the break down of urine.

narcissism – an abnormal mental state where there is excessive admiration of oneself.

narcolepsy – a condition characterised by sudden uncontrollable attacks of deep sleep, during waking hours, sometimes occurring 2–3 times a day.

narcosis – profound insensibility resembling deep sleep with the individual only rousable by great efforts. Most commonly the condition is caused by drugs.

nausea – a feeling that vomiting is about to take place.

neoplasm – any abnormal new growth either benign or malignant.

nephritis – any of various acute or chronic inflammatory conditions of the kidney. When chronic it is also known as Bright's disease.

RICHARD BRIGHT (1789 – 1858) who was born in Bristol was the first physician to describe the clinical manifestations of the kidney disorder nephritis, which became known as Bright's disease. He graduated in medicine from Edinburgh and later became assistant physician at Guy's Hospital in 1820 and full physician in 1825. It was in his 'Reports of Medical Cases' published in 1827 that he established that oedema and proteinuria were the principal features of the disorder carrying his name.

nephroblastoma – see Wilm's tumour.

nephrolithiasis – a condition in which calculi are present in the kidney(s).

nephroptosis – movable or floating kidney.

nephrostomy – making an opening into the kidney to drain it.

nephrotic syndrome – a condition associated with hyperalbuminuria whereby the albumen leaks through the glomerulus and gross oedema. Normally the result of primary renal disease. The condition may be the result of auto-immune disease such as systemic lupus erythematosus or metabolic diseases such as diabetes or amyloidosis or due to malignant disease. It is often the end result of kidney failure.

nettle rash – another term for urticaria.

> **neurasthenia** – a condition of nervous exhaustion where there are no definite signs of disease. The individual is incapable of sustained activity.

neuritis – inflammation affecting a nerve or nerves of the body. It may be caused by compression, infection, toxins, drugs and other causes.

neurodermatitis – a disease of the skin in which stress is one if not the most important factor such as pruritis, rosacea and to a lesser extent atopic eczema and lichen simplex.

neurofibromatosis – another name for von Recklinghausen's disease.

> Neurofibromatosis can sometimes result in gross disfiguration. This effect came to public attention with the Broadway play in the early 80s, the Elephant Man, which was the true story of a young Englishman who was presumed to have been deformed by the disease. The play was later made into a film, which starred the actor, John Hurt.

neuroma – a tumour made up of nervous and its accompanying fibrous tissue. It may be painful.

neuromyaesthenia – a condition which occurs in epidemics characterised by headaches, stiffness of the neck and back, pain, fever and diarrhoea. It may be caused by a virus or hysteria. It is sometimes referred to as Royal Free disease because of an epidemic in that hospital a few years ago.

neurosis – any of various illnesses affecting the mind or emotions without obvious organic lesion or change. It involves anxiety, depression, phobia, hysteria or other abnormal patterns of behaviour. There is no serious disturbance in perception or understanding of external reality as in the psychoses.

neurotic – a general term of indefinite meaning applied to persons of nervous temperament whose actions are largely determined by emotion or instinct rather than reason.

neutropenia – a reduction in the number of neutrophils in the blood. It can be a feature of conditions such as typhoid, influenza or due to some drugs.

Nieman-Pick disease – a rare hereditary condition occurring almost exclusively in children of Jewish families. It is a disorder of fat metabolism which goes on to produce anaemia, emaciation, mental retardation, blindness and deafness. Affected children rarely survive after their second year.

night blindness – the inability to see in the dark. It is usually associated with retinitis pigmentosa or vitamin A deficiency.

night sweats – copious perspiration occurring in bed at night sometimes associated with tuberculosis, brucellosis or lymphosarcoma.

nocturia – excess passing of urine during the night; can be associated with glomerulonephritis and prostate enlargement.

nocturnal enuresis – involuntary passing of urine in one's sleep (bedwetting). It occurs predominantly in children and only a few cases have an organic cause.

noma – another name for cancrum oris, a condition characterised by ulcers around the mouth which lead to gangrene, occurring in children.

non-specific urethritis – inflammation of the urethra due to a number of different organisms e.g. chlamydia, the commonest sexually transmitted disease. It is not caused by the gonococcus or any of the more easily identifiable specific organisms.

Norwegian scabies – a rare form of scabies, found in Scotland, which is severe and in which the skin becomes greatly thickened and fissures develop.

nosophobe – a person who has a morbid fear of contracting a certain disease.

nostalgia – a form of melancholy or aggravated home sickness in persons who have left their homes.

nyctalopia – a technical term for night blindness.

nymphomania – an excessive sexual desire in a woman.

nystagmus – a spasmodic involuntary rhythmic oscillation of the eyeballs either horizontally, vertically or rotatory. It may indicate a disturbance of the inner ear or a disorder of the central nervous system.

obesity – a condition of the body characterised by over-accumulation of fat under the skin and around certain internal organs.

ochronosis – a rare condition in which the ligaments and cartilages of the body and sometimes the conjunctiva become stained by dark brown or black pigment. It may occur in chronic carbolic poisoning or in the congenital disorder of metabolism, alkaptanuria, whereby the body is unable to break up completely the tyrosine of the protein molecule.

oedema – an abnormal accumulation of fluid beneath the skin and in the cavities of the body.

oedema of the lungs – an accumulation of fluid in the lungs most often the result of the left ventricle being unable to handle the blood delivered to it; it occurs as a result of myocardial infarction and other causes of left ventricular failure such as hypertension and valvular disease.

oesophagitis – inflammation of the lining of the oesophagus.

oligaemia – a diminution of the quantity of blood in circulation.

oligomenhorrhoea – scanty menstruation or an abnormally long time between menstrual periods.

oligophrenia – mental deficiency, feeble mindedness.

oligospermia – abnormally few spermatozoa in the semen.

oliguria – abnormally low excretion of urine.

omphalocoele – another name for examphalos, the herniation of abdominal organs through the umbilicus.

> **onchocerciasis** – infestation with the filarial worm Onchocerca volvulus, occurring in tropical Africa, south of the Sahara, Central and South America, Yemen and Saudi Arabia. The infection with the threadlike worms produces tumours in the skin and sometimes a blinding disease of the eyes.

onychia – inflammation affecting the nails.

onychogryphosis – a distortion of the nail which becomes thickened and overgrown, twisted on itself. It usually affects the toenail and is the result of chronic irritation and inflammation.

onycholysis – a separation of the nail from the nail bed.

oophoritis – another name for inflammation of the ovary.

ophthalmia – inflammation of the eye, a term sometimes used instead of conjunctivitis.

ophthalmoplegia – paralysis of the muscle of the eye.

opisthotonos – a position assumed by the body during one of the convulsive attacks of tetanus. The muscle of the back arches the body in such a way that the person for a time rests upon the heels and the head.

orchidectomy – an operation for the removal of one or both the testicles.

orchidopexy – an operation to bring the testes into the scrotum in those with undescended testicles.

orchitis – inflammation of the testicles.

orf – a viral infection of sheep and goats, sometimes affecting man. It is characterised by a skin eruption usually on the hands, fingers, forearms and face.

oriental sore – single or multiple skin ulcers produced by an infection spread by sandflies. It is otherwise known as cutaneous Leishmaniasis. Delhi boil or Aleppo evil.

ornithosis – a pneumonia-like disease produced by viruses from infected birds. The organism involved is Chlamydia psittacosis.

orthopnoea – difficulty in breathing so severe that the patient cannot breathe lying down so that he has to sit or stand up; it usually only occurs in those with serious affections of the heart and lungs.

Osgood–Schlatter's disease – osteochondritis of the tibial tubercle. It occurs mainly around puberty as a painful swelling which is worse after exertion.

osteitis – inflammation in the substance of the bone.

osteitis deformans – a chronic condition of bone overgrowth, destruction and new bone formation all producing deformities. The skull, spine and weight bearing bones are most commonly affected; it is otherwise known as Paget's disease.

osteitis fibrosa – a condition where the bone is replaced by highly cellular and vascular connective tissue. The condition is caused by excessive parathyroid activity and uraemic osteodystrophy (secondary hyperparathyroidism occurring in patients with chronic renal disease).

osteoarthrosis (itis) – a chronic degeneration of the bone end composing a joint and leading to deformity.

osteochondritis – inflammation of both bone and cartilage. It may be a common cause of backache in young people.

osteochondrosis – a group of disease involving the degeneration of the centres of ossification in the growing bones of children e.g. Kohler's disease, Osgood-Schlatter's and Perthé's disease.

osteogenesis imperfecta – a rare hereditary condition of defective formation of bony tissue resulting in brittle bones which fracture easily.

osteomalacia – an adult form of rickets involving a softening of the bones, abnormal flexibility, brittleness, loss of calcium salts. It is usually due to vitamin D deficiency or impaired absorption of nutrients.

osteomyelitis – an inflammation of the bone and marrow due to growth of organisms within the bone. Infection may also affect the bloodstream.

> **osteoporosis** – brittleness and increased porousness of the bones resulting in a liability to fracture. It is common in elderly people, particularly in women after the menopause.

osteosarcoma – the most common and most malignant tumour of bone. It usually occurs in the ends of the long bones in older children and young adults.

otalgia – earache.

otitis – inflammation of the ear. Otitis externa is a bacterial or fungal infection of the ear canal. Otitis media is an acute or chronic infection (usually bacterial) of the middle ear.

otomycosis – an infection of the external ear by a fungus such as aspergillus or candida.

otorrhoea – chronic discharge from the ear.

Father of Gynaecology

A small pair of obstetric forceps called Wrigley's Forceps, still in use for infant delivery, were named after their inventor Joseph Wrigley, an eminent obstetrician who was still practising when the compiler was a student.

A friend of the compiler, sitting his finals' viva in obstetrics, was presented with a pair of these forceps by the examiner with the question: "Which forceps are these?" "Wrigley's forceps, sir," came the reply. "Who is or was Wrigley?" pursued the examiner. Confusing Wrigley with another eminent obstetrician and gynaecologist of a previous age, the compiler's friend replied: "He was the father of gynaecology, sir."

The examiner rose from his chair, went over to the next table where Wrigley was an examiner, put his hand on his shoulder, pointed to the student and said: "He says you're the father of gynaecology!"

Joe Wrigley's comment was not recorded!

---

otosclerosis – abnormal bone deposited by the footplate of the stapes producing conductive deafness. The abnormal bone dampens vibrations which impairs hearing. This type of deafness can be corrected by surgery.

ovarian cyst – a sac containing fluid or mucoid material arising in the ovary.

overlaying of infants – a process whereby an infant sleeping in the same bed as an adult is suffocated as a result of the adult lying on top of the infant.

oxycephaly – otherwise known as steeple head. It is a deformity of the skull in which the forehead bulge is high and the top of the head is parted. There is also poor vision and the eyes bulge.

oxyuris – another name for threadworms.

ozaena – a chronic disease of the mucous membranes of the nose giving off foul smelling odour or discharge.

pachyderma – hypertrophy or thickening of the skin.

pachyderma laryngis – thickness of the vocal cords due to chronic inflammation or irritation.

pachymeningitis – inflammation of the dura mater of the brain and spinal cord.

> SIR JAMES PAGET (1814-1899), a British Surgeon and Physiologist, is considered to be one of the founders of the science of pathology.
>
> He was Professor of Surgery and Anatomy at St. Bartholomew's Hospital and became President of the Royal College of Surgeons in 1871.
>
> He gave an excellent description of breast cancer, an early indication of which became known as Paget's disease of the nipple and he also described Paget's disease of bone.
>
> He was one of the first to recommend surgical removal of bone marrow tumours (myeloid sarcoma) instead of amputation of the limb.

Paget's disease of the breast – the condition is manifested by thickened eczema-like scaliness of the area around the nipple with fissure formation, a discharge and destruction of the nipple as the disease progresses. The underlying disease process is cancer of the central ducts of the breast.

Paget's disease of bone – see osteitis deformans.

painter's colic – abdominal colic due to lead poisoning.

palindromic rheumatism – multiple afebrile attacks of acute arthritis with inflammation of surrounding tissue, characterised by pain, swelling, redness and disability in one or more joints and occurring in adults.

palpitation – a condition in which the heart beats forcibly or irregularly and the person becomes conscious of its action.

palsy – another name for paralysis.

pancarditis – inflammation of the pericardium, myocardium and endocardium at the same time.

pancreatitis – inflammation of the pancreas which can be in an acute or chronic form. The former causes acute pain, shock and sometimes collapse, while in the chronic form it can be due to conditions of the gall bladder and chronic alcoholism.

panhypopituitarism – a severe loss of function of the anterior pituitary gland.

panniculitis – inflammation of the sub-cutaneous fat.

panophthalmitis – a pus producing inflammation of all the tissues of the eye which can give rise to total and permanent blindness.

papillitis – inflammation of papillae especially of the prominences found by the end of the optic nerve in the retina, which is known as optic neuritis.

> **papilloedema** – a swelling of the optic disc due to raised intracranial pressure. It occurs most frequently in patients with a brain tumour, brain abscess, meningitis, concussion, haemorrhage or severe hypertension.

papilloma – a tumour lining tissues such as skin, mucous membranes and glandular ducts. They are usually benign but they can become malignant. In the bladder they can produce bleeding giving rise to haematuria.

papovirus – group of viruses responsible for warts.

papule – another term for pimple.

paracusis – any perversion of the sense of hearing.

paraesthesia – unusual feelings of loss of sensation without necessarily an established cause. The sensations can be of crawling, burning or tingling of the skin which may be due to neuritis or other lesions of the nervous system.

paraganglioma – a term for two types of tumour, chromaffinoma or phaeochromocytoma which are tumours of the chromaffin cells of the adrenal medulla producing severe hypertension and chromodectoma, a small tumour in the carotid body and in the comparable small aortic area.

paragonimiasis – an infestation by the trematode or fluke Paragonima westermani which can be found in the Far East, India and Africa. The worms enter the lungs causing haemoptysis. It is acquired by eating inadequately cooked crayfish or crabs.

paragraphia – the writing of words or letters other than those intended or an inability to express ideas in writing. Can result from certain disorders of the brain.

paralysis – a loss of muscular power due to interference with the nervous system. Also known as palsy.

paralytic ileus – intestinal obstruction due to decreased peristalsis in the bowel.

parametritis – inflammation of the cellular tissue at the side of the womb.

paramnesia – a derangement of the memory involving the use of words without a comprehension of their meaning. It is also an illness of memory in which the person, in good faith, imagines and describes experiences which never occurred to him or her.

paramyoclonus – paroxysmal jerky contractions of the muscles of the limb sometimes due to organic disease of the nervous system or sometimes due to hysteria.

paranoia – a mental illness manifested by fixed delusions usually of persecution. Many sufferers can go about freely and carry out activities with which their delusions do not interfere.

paraphasia – a misplacement of words or use of wrong words due to a lesion in the specific speech area of the brain.

paraphrenia – a form of paranoia.

paraplegia – paralysis of the lower limbs and usually associated with paralysis of the bladder and rectum.

parasuicide – non-fatal self poisoning or attempted suicide; sometimes referred to as 'a cry for help'.

paratyphoid – an acute infection which resembles typhoid but is less severe. It is caused by the Salmonella paratyphi group of bacteria.

paresis – a state of partial paralysis.

Parkinson's disease – sometimes known as paralysis agitans. It is a progressive disease of insidious onset occurring in the second half of life with degenerative changes in the ganglia at the base of the cerebrum. This causes a deficiency in the neurotransmitter chemical, dopamine. It occurs in men more frequently than women and is sometimes a sequel to encephalitis lethergica (sleepy sickness). It is characterised by an increasing rigidity of the muscles, a mask-like expression, a tremor, particularly in the hands, flat voice and a characteristic gait where the patient appears to be 'catching up with himself'.

paronychia – an infection near the nail usually due to a staphylococcus or a fungus.

parosmia – a perverted sense of smell.

parotitis – an inflammation of the parotid gland. In its epidemic form it is known as mumps.

paroxysmal tachycardia – periodic attacks of rapid beating of the heart lasting a few seconds or as long as several hours.

parulis – a gumboil or an abscess of the gum.

Patterson-Kelly syndrome – see Plummer-Vinson syndrome.

pediculosis – infestation with lice on the head, body or pubis.

pellagra – a nutritional disorder producing nervous, digestive and skin symptoms. It can be characterised by dermatitis, diarrhoea and dementia. It is caused by a deficiency of vitamin B3 nicotinic acid.

pemphigus – an uncommon but serious skin disease manifested by crops of large blisters which rupture and produce raw areas. It is regarded as an auto-immune disease.

PENICILLIN

Millions of people who have suffered from a variety of infections have cause to be grateful to the Scottish bacteriologist, Sir Alexander Fleming (1881-1955).

In 1928, working in his laboratory at St. Mary's Hospital, Paddington, he noted a bacteria free circle around a mould (Penicillium notatum) which had contaminated one of his bacterial cultures. He found a substance in this mould which he called penicillin and which prevented the growth of staphylococci.

This work was carried forwards by Ernst Chain and Howard Florey, at Oxford's William Dunn laboratory. They succeeded in the isolation, purification, testing and the production of penicillin.

Due to the war it was not possible to produce the antibiotic in sufficient quantities, so its manufacture was taken over by a number of American pharmaceutical companies.

peptic ulcer – an ulcer in the stomach or duodenum associated with the digestive action of the juices.

perforation – one of a series of dangers and complications associated with ulcerative conditions of the stomach or bowels.

pericarditis – inflammation of the pericardium (the sac of fibrous tissue surrounding the heart).

perimetritis – localised inflammation of the peritoneum surrounding the womb.

periodic paralysis – characterised by the onset of weakness of the voluntary muscles occurring in young adults. The onset takes place in the morning on awakening.

periodontal disease – inflammation of the membranes covering the roots of the teeth, commonly called pyorrhoea.

periostitis – inflammation of the surface of the bone affecting the periosteum.

peripheral neuritis – inflammation of the nerves in the outlying parts of the body.

peritonitis – inflammation of the peritoneum or membranes investing the abdominal and pelvic cavities and the visceral organs they contain. In its acute form it can be due the bursting of an inflamed organ or a perforation. In a chronic form it can be due to tuberculosis.

peritonsillar abscess – a collection of pus between the tonsil and the superior constrictor muscle of the pharynx. It is a complication of tonsillitis; also known as a quinsy.

pernicious anaemia – an auto-immune disease whereby sensitised lymphocytes destroy the parietal cells of the stomach which normally produce the intrinsic factor, the carrier protein for vitamin B_{12} that permits its absorption in the terminal ileum. If vitamin B_{12} is not absorbed it gives rise to macrocytic anaemia. The skin and mucosa become pale and the tongue becomes smooth and atrophic. It can present as peripheral neuropathy with paraesthesia and numbness. It can proceed to the neurological complication, subacute combined degeneration of the cord. The condition is easily treatable by injections of vitamin B_{12}.

THOMAS ADDISON (1793-1860) – born in Lowbrunton, Northumberland.

In 1837 he became a physician at Guy's Hospital and joint lecturer with Richard Bright.

He was the first to correlate a set of disease symptoms with pathological changes in one of the endocrine glands. He was also the first to describe pernicious anaemia.

Apart from his other writings he wrote an essay on 'The operation of poisonous agents upon the living body'.

Perhaps it is appropriate that today, Guy's Hospital has one of the most noted poisons unit in the country.

perseveration – senseless repetition of words and deeds in persons with a disordered mind.

Perthé's disease – the condition is due to osteochondritis of the head of the femur causing degeneration of the hip in children usually between the ages of 4-20, affecting boys ten times as frequently as girls.

pertussis – another name for whooping cough.

pes cavus – another name for flat feet.

pest – another name for plague.

petechiae – small spots on the skin of a red/purple colour, like flea bites. They are due to small haemorrhages under the skin.

petit mal – a lesser type of epileptic seizure, usually occurring in children, whereby there is a sudden loss of consciousness lasting a few seconds. Nowadays the attacks are referred to as 'absence' attacks.

phagedaena – an ulcer of the skin and subcutaneous tissues that spreads rapidly and causes sloughing off of the skin.

phantasy – imaginary appearance or a day dream.

phantom limb – following amputation the patient experiences sensations as if the limb were still present. It usually passes off with time.

pharyngitis – inflammation of the wall of the pharynx usually due to a virus infection.

> **phenylketonuria** – hereditary inability to metabolize phenylalanine, an essential aminoacid, due to the lack of the necessary enzyme. The breakdown products of incompletely metabolised phenylalanine accumulate in the body of the infant causing impairment of the infant's brain function giving rise to a severe form of mental deficiency. The condition can easily be detected by a blood test early in infancy and the sequelae can be prevented by the administration of a diet low in phenylalanine.

phimosis – tightness of the foreskin of the penis making retraction over the tip of the penis very difficult.

phlebitis – inflammation of the walls of a vein which may give rise to clot formation; it occurs most commonly in the leg veins but it can occur in other veins particularly in the arms after intravenous injections.

phlebolith – a small stone found in a vein as a result of the calcification of a clot.

phlebothrombosis – the formation of a clot in a vein but not necessarily due to local inflammation.

phlegm – a popular name for mucus particularly that secreted in the air passages.

phlegmasia dolens – another name for white leg.

phlyctenule – hypersensitivity reaction of the conjunctiva to a staphylococcus or tuberculosis.

phobia – irrational fear of objects or situations.

phocomelia – a great reduction in size of the proximal parts of the limbs.

phosphaturia – the presence of large amounts of phosphates in the urine.

phosphorus poisoning – produced by the yellow soluble form of phosphorus e.g. by swallowing rat poison. It firstly causes irritation in the stomach then, after absorption, degenerative changes occur in the liver and other organs. There can also be chronic exposure to fumes in chemical workers causing profound disability and disease in the lower jaw (phossy jaw) which necroses and bits come away in large fragments.

> **photodermatosis (itis)** – eruptions on areas of skin exposed to sunlight; the condition can be exacerbated by certain drugs e.g. chlorpromazine.

photophobia – sensitivity of the eyes to light which can be due to disorders of the eye or meningitis.

phthiriasis – a condition consisting of eczema, matted hair, dirt and enlarged glands due to the crab louse.

phthisis – wasting, progressive weakness and loss of weight arising from tuberculosis, particularly of the lungs.

pica – an abnormal craving for unusual foods e.g. as in pregnancy.

pigeon breeder's lung – see bird fancier's lung.

piles – see haemorrhoids.

pimples – another name for papules; small round inflamed areas of skin.

pink disease – see erythroedema.

pink eye – an obsolete term to describe a highly infectious, usually viral, disease of the conjunctiva.

pins and needles – a form of paraesthesia, neuritis or polyneuritis.

> **pithiatism** – a group of diseases in which patients are subject to cure by persuasion or suggestion e.g. hysteria.

pituitary cachexia – see Simmond's disease.

pityriasis alba – a form of chronic eczema occurring mainly in children. It is characterised by rounded scaly white patches usually on the face but sometimes on the upper arms or back. The condition is self limiting but may drag on for several years.

pityriasis rosea – a non-infectious and non-contagious skin disease of young adults characterised by scaly patches. The condition starts with the appearance of an oval, slightly red, scaly area between the shoulders or on the lower abdomen (herald patch) 3-4 days before the main eruption. The condition lasts for 6 weeks and does not recur.

placenta praevia – the placenta develops in the lower part of the uterus sometimes over the opening of the cervix. It is one of the causes of bleeding during pregnancy.

plagiocephaly – a congenital abnormality of the skull with flattening of the forehead on one side of the skull and bossing or bulging on the other.

plague – another name for bubonic plague.

plantar dermatosis – cracks and fissures in the skin on the soles of the feet occurring in children.

plaque – a coating occurring on the teeth as a result of neglect.

plethora – a condition of fullness of the blood vessels in a particular part of the body. The volume of blood in those areas is increased above normal.

pleurisy – inflammation of the pleura causing sharp pains aggravated by deep breathing or coughing. There are wet or dry forms of the condition.

pleurodynia – a sharp pain in the muscles between the ribs. It is characteristic of Bornholm disease (qv).

pleuro-pneumonia – a combination of pleurisy with pneumonia. Pneumonia is usually accompanied by some degree of pleurisy but the epidemic disease known as pleuro-pneumonia is restricted to horned cattle and does not occur in man.

plumbism – another name for lead poisoning.

> **Plummer-Vinson syndrome** – a condition associated with hypochromic anaemia characterised by difficulty in swallowing, particularly in women. Otherwise known as the Patterson-Kelly syndrome.

pneumoconiosis – a general name applied to a chronic form of inflammation of the lungs liable to affect workmen constantly inhaling irritating particles at work.

pneumonectomy – removal of a whole lung.

pneumonia – inflammation of the lung caused by various organisms. The inflammation is in the lung substance and is associated with consolidation, the lung tissue becoming solid and airless. It can be classified according to the anatomical part affected e.g. lobar, segmental, bronchopneumonia.

pneumonitis – inflammation of the lung due to chemical or physical agents.

pneumoperitoneum – a collection of air in the peritoneum sometimes carried out deliberately to collapse a lung.

pneumothorax – a collection of air in the pleural cavity which gains entry by a lesion in the lung or chest wall. As a result the lung collapses. After the air is removed or is absorbed the lung re-expands.

podagra – another name for gout.

poikilocytosis – describes the variations seen in shapes of blood cells in some bone marrow disorders.

> **policeman's heel** – caused by walking on the foot, often occurring in obesity. It is a form of fasciitis and can give rise to a calcaneal spur. It is a painful condition and is worse after rest. It can be relieved by the use of a sorbo rubber pad.

poliomyelitis – an infectious disease affecting the spinal cord and brain, due to a virus. The virus is ingested through the mouth. The motor cells in the anterior horns of the spinal cord are affected with a greater tendency to affect the lumbar region. The cranial nerves can also be involved. The incubation period is 3-21 days. The most severe form can also cause paralysis of the muscles of the diaphragm. Immunisation gives a high degree of protection.

poliosis – premature greying of the hair.

polyarteritis nodosa – a rare disease characterised by inflammation and nodular swellings of the artery walls sometimes leading to the death of local tissue. The condition is classified as a disorder of connective tissue.

polychromasia (polychromatophilia) – an abnormal reaction of red blood cells in severe anaemia. After removal of a sample the blood cells develop a bluish tinge on standing. This is a sign that the cells are not fully developed.

polycystic kidneys – a congenital defect in which the kidneys are filled with bubble-like cysts.

polycystic ovary syndrome – a condition of the ovaries in which the women affected present with hirsutism, infertility, oligomenorrhoea or amenhorroea.

polycythaemia – a condition characterised by an abnormal increase in haemoglobin concentration and the number of red blood cells. The primary variety (polycythaemia rubra vera) is of unknown cause and is accompanied by a grossly enlarged spleen. The condition can be secondary to tissue hypoxia, as a compensatory mechanism.

BEST LAID PLANS?

Clinical trials with a new treatment often involve the double-blind technique so that neither the patient nor the physician knows which treatment the patient is taking.

Some years ago a new injectable drug was being tried in schizophrenic in-patients. Half the patients received the new injection and dummy chlorpromazine tablets and the other half dummy injections and active chlorpromazine, a standard drug used to treat schizophrenia.

All went well until one sunny day all the patients decided to sunbathe. Chlorpromazine is known to cause photosensitivity and the patients taking that treatment all came out in a rash so everyone knew which patients were in which group!

polydactyly – the presence of extra supernumerary fingers or toes.

polydipsia – the presence of excessive thirst, which is a manifestation of diabetes mellitus or diabetes insipidus.

polymorphic light eruption – a photodermatosis predominantly in women made up of a mixture of erythema, papules and vesicles on parts of the body exposed to the sun. There are usually several attacks a year depending on the amount of sun. Although produced by sunlight the underlying cause is unknown.

polymyalgia rheumatica – a form of rheumatism characterised by gross early morning stiffness easing as the day progresses. The pain is principally in the shoulders and sometimes in the limbs. It occurs in women 60 times more frequently than in men. The cause is obscure.

polyneuritis – an inflammatory condition of the nerves of various parts of the body.

polyposis – the presence of a crop or large number of polyps. The most important variety occurs in the large bowel which is a familial condition in which the polyps can undergo cancerous change.

polypi (polyps) – tumours attached by a stalk to the surface from which they spring.

polythelia – extra or supernumerary nipples appearing along a line between the armpit and the groin.

polyuria – the passage of an excessive amount of urine, a symptom of diabetes mellitus, diabetes insipidus, renal failure or of a psychogenic cause.

pompholyx – a form of eczema characterised by the appearance of deeply set vesicles on the side of the fingers or toes.

porencephaly – a term applied to the presence of cysts in the surface of the brain due to an arrest of development or haemorrhage at birth. It gives rise to serious mental defects.

> **porphyria** – a condition characterised by the excessive excretion of porphyrins in the urine. Porphyrins are a constituent of various blood and respiratory pigments found throughout the animal kingdom including man. The disturbance of metabolism leads to discolouration of urine, skin rashes due to the sensitivity of the skin to light, various forms of indigestion and mental disturbance. Porphyria is believed to be responsible for the insanity of George III.

porrigo – a general term applied to diseases of the skin of the head such as ringworm.

post–viral fatigue syndrome – a condition following a virus infection where the patient suffers from physical exhaustion, disability and incapacity. Recent evidence suggests that it is due to an enterovirus such as coxsachie B but other viruses may be involved. It is sometimes referred to as ME (myeloencephalopathy).

Pott's disease – an angular curvature of the spine resulting from tuberculosis.

Pott's fracture – a variety of fracture around the ankle. The fibula is fractured in all cases with a varying degree of dislocation. It is often mistaken for a sprain.

pre-eclampsia – a complication of pregnancy characterised by oedema, high blood pressure and albuminuria. If untreated it may proceed to eclampsia.

premenstrual syndrome – cyclic occurrence of emotional symptoms associated with body changes about a week before the onset of a menstrual period.

presbycusis – deafness which comes on after increasing years. It is due to loss of elasticity in the hearing mechanism with the slowing down of mental processes, accompanying old age.

presbyopia – the change in eyesight caused by ageing requiring the wearing of glasses for close vision.

pressure sores – see bedsores.

prickly heat – a troublesome skin condition affecting Europeans in tropical climates. It is characterised by vesicles due to the blocking of the outlet of sweat or sebaceous glands and giving rise to severe itching.

procidentia – another name for a prolapse.

proctalgia – neuralgic pain in the rectum or anus. The term usually refers to rectal pain without local disease to account for it. Proctalgia fugax is a condition where there is excruciating pain occurring in the night lasting up to 15 minutes and is more common in women.

proctitis – inflammation in the rectum or anus.

prodromata – the earliest symptoms of a disease.

progeria – premature old age.

progressive muscular atrophy – a form of motor neurone disease. There is a long delay before the wasting of the hand muscles begin to spread to other parts.

prolapse – the slipping down of some organs or structure.

prolapsed intervertebral disc – the centre of the disc herniates out exerting pressure on the adjacent spinal nerves. It most commonly occurs in the discs between the lumbar vertebrae.

proptosis – a condition in which the eyes protrude from the orbit e.g. in thyroid disease.

prostatism – a condition caused by benign enlargement of the prostate.

prostatitis – acute or chronic inflammation of the prostate.

prosthesis – an artificial replacement such as of a limb, eye, denture or breast.

proteinuria – the presence of protein (usually albumen) in the urine.

prurigo – a chronic skin disease characterised by small papules and severe itching.

pruritis – another name for itching.

prussic acid poisoning – the condition is characterised by shortness of breath, heart irregularities, blueness of the face and lips and convulsions usually leading to death. It is the same as cyanide poisoning and may be detected by the smell of bitter almonds.

pseudocyesis – false or phantom pregnancy.

pseudohypertrophic muscular dystrophy – the muscles enlarge due to fibrous and fatty degeneration giving a false impression of increased strength.

pseudoxanthoma elastica – a hereditary disorder of elastic tissue. The degeneration produces lesions in the skin like soft yellow papules also affecting the eyes and blood vessels causing visual impairment, raised blood pressure and haemorrhages.

psitticosis – a pneumonia-like disease transmitted by infected birds. The disease not only affects birds of the parrot family but also pigeons, chickens, ducks, turkeys and other birds.

psoriasis – a chronic disease of the skin of unknown cause, usually persisting for years with periods of remission and recurrence. It is characterised by elevated lesions on various parts of the body such as the elbows, knees, scalp, nails and lower back, which are covered with silvery scales. General health is rarely affected but psoriatic arthropathy, a form of arthritis in the fingers and toes, can develop in some sufferers.

psychoneurosis – a general term applied to various functional diseases of the nervous system. The condition is an emotionally based disturbance of the personality severe enough to be handicapping.

psychopathy – a personality disorder of the mind characterised by aggression or social irresponsibility. The psychopath cannot learn from experience, lacks moral judgement and cannot form stable relationships.

psychosomatic disease – a disease sometimes, but not always without accompanying physical cause.

pterygium – degenerative condition affecting the conjunctiva which grows over the cornea both medially and laterally. The overgrowths present a wing-like appearance.

ptyalism – excess production of saliva.

puerperal fever – an infection occurring in the puerperium after pregnancy caused by the haemolytic streptococcus.

pulmonary embolism – a clot lodged in the lungs, sometimes a serious complication after surgery.

purpura – a condition in which bleeding occurs in the skin or mucous membranes due to a deficiency of blood platelets.

pustule – small collection of pus.

putrid fever – an old name for typhoid.

pyaemia – a form of blood poisoning in which abscesses appear in parts of the body.

pyelitis – also known as pyelo-nephritis, whereby the pelvis of the kidney becomes infected, most commonly by the bacterial organism Escherichia coli.

pyknolepsy – a type of epilepsy where the only manifestation is a sudden and temporary loss of consciousness with no convulsions.

pyelophlebitis – inflammation of the portal vein; usually a part of general blood poisoning.

pylorospasm – a spasm of the muscle at the outlet of the stomach. The condition is painful and occurs 1/2 -3 hours after a meal.

pyloric stenosis – obstruction of the outlet of the stomach. It can occur as a complication of chronic peptic ulceration or in babies due to a thickening of the pyloric muscle encircling the pylorus.

pyoderma gangrenosum – a condition in which large ulcerated lesions appear suddenly on the skin. There is an underlying vasculitis as a result of inflammatory bowel disease or rheumatoid arthritis.

pyorrhoea – means a copious flow of pus; it is commonly used as the name for a disease of the gums, periodontoclasia, which is an inflammation and gradual destruction of the supporting tissues of the teeth.

pyrexia – another name for fever.

pyrosis – a symptom of dyspepsia when the mouth fills with tasteless or sour fluid from the stomach (waterbrash).

pyuria – the presence of pus in the urine

Q fever – a self-limiting disease caused by the rickettsial organism, Coxiella burnetti, resembling pneumonia. It is a worldwide disease first described in 1937 among abattoir workers in Brisbane.

quadrantopia – inability to be able to see in one quarter of the visual field; homonymous quadrantopia is the loss of vision in the same quarter of each eye.

quadriplegia – paralysis of both arms and both legs.

quartan fever – intermittent feverish paroxysms every fourth day (applied to malaria).

quinsy – an old name for an abscess around the tonsil (peritonsillar abscess).

rabies – an acute and fatal viral disease affecting animals (particularly carnivores), which can be communicated to man. It affects the central nervous system and is characterised by convulsions and aversion to water (hydrophobia). It has an incubation period of one month to a year or more. If a human is bitten by a rabid animal prompt injections of rabies vaccine can prevent the disease from taking hold. The disease is rare in the U.K. due to strict quarantine regulations.

LOUIS PASTEUR (1822-1895) was a French microbiologist and chemist. He is recognised as the founder of modern microbiology who became professor at the Sorbonne in 1867. He discovered that micro-organisms in the air were responsible for the fermentation of beer and milk. In his investigations into ways of excluding these organisms he developed the process of pasteurisation, which is responsible for the elimination of tuberculosis organisms from milk. Pasteur also developed vaccines for anthrax, chicken cholera and, most importantly, rabies.

radiation sickness – nausea, vomiting and loss of appetite following the use of radiotherapy.

ranula – a swelling occasionally appearing under the tongue. It is made up of a collection of saliva in a distended duct of a salivary gland.

rat-bite fever – an infectious disease following the bite of a rat. There are two different diseases: one caused by Spirillus minus with ulceration at the site of the bite, a purplish rash and recurrent fever. The other is caused by Actinobacillus muris and characterised by skin inflammation, back and joint pains, headache and vomiting. Both can be treated with penicillin.

Raynaud's disease – first described by Maurice Raynaud in 1862. The circulation becomes obstructed in the outlying parts of the body, probably due to spasms of the small arteries of the affected part causing pallor and numbness. The effect is increased by coldness and various diseases affecting the blood vessels. The condition is commonest in women before the age of 40 causing 'dead' fingers. In its severest form Raynaud's disease can lead to gangrene of the fingers.

reactive arthritis – aseptic arthritis following an episode of infection elsewhere in the body. It can occur following salmonella or shigella infections. Non-gonococcal arthritis is one of the signs of Reiter's syndrome.

recrudescence – the reappearance of a disease after a period without signs or symptoms of its presence.

rectocoele – bulging of the rectum through the rear wall of the vagina.

red gum – see strophulus.

referred pain – pain felt in one part of the body which actually arises from a distant site e.g. pain in or near the diaphragm is often referred to the shoulder tip. It usually occurs because the sites are developed from similar embryonic tissue having common pain pathways in the central nervous system.

reflux – fluid flowing in the opposite direction to normal. It often refers to regurgitation of the stomach contents into the oesophagus.

regional ileitis – another name for Crohn's disease.

Reiter's syndrome – a condition characterised by arthritis, urethritis (non-gonococcal) and conjunctivitis. It can arise from promiscuous sexual contact or follow an unrelated gastro-intestinal infection with Yersinia enterocolitica.

rejection – the body's immunological response to foreign tissue.

relapse – the return of a disease during convalescence.

relapsing fever – a condition producing a characteristic temperature chart with recurring bouts of fever. It is caused by spirochaetes. The louse-borne spirochaete Borrelia recurrentis occurs in epidemics. The tick-borne variety caused by Borrelia duboni is endemic in most tropical and sub-tropical areas. In this latter form there is a shorter incubation period with shorter febrile periods but with relapses more common.

remittent fever – a form of fever which, during remission, the temperature falls but not to normal.

remission – a period when a disease has responded to treatment with no symptoms or signs present.

repetitive strain injury – tendonitis caused by the constant use of a keyboard, occurring in the hands and arms.

respiratory distress syndrome – another name for hyaline membrane disease.

> **restless legs syndrome** – the experience of unpleasant sensations and involuntary movements of the legs at rest, particularly at night.

retardation – slowing down or developmental delay.

retention of urine – urine, secreted by the kidney, is retained in the bladder. This can be due to some physical obstruction, as in prostatic enlargement, or due to interference with the control of micturition, as in some neurological diseases.

> **reticulosis** – a condition characterised by progressive widespread proliferation of the cells of the reticuloendothelial system as in Hodgkin's disease and lymphosarcoma.

retinopathy – a disease or abnormality in the retina.

retinitis pigmentosa – hereditary degeneration and atrophy of the retina.

retinoblastoma – a malignant tumour of the retina which is an inherited condition occurring in infants and young children.

retrobulbar neuritis – an inflammation of the optic nerve behind the eye. It is a condition of young adults causing rapid deterioration of vision including coloured vision. It usually lasts only a few weeks. The condition sometimes follows a virus illness or it may occur in patients with multiple sclerosis.

retropharyngeal abscess – an abscess in the cellular tissue behind the throat as a result, generally, of disease in the upper part of the spinal column.

retroversion – abnormal position of the uterus.

> **Reye's syndrome** – a condition occurring predominantly in young children following an upper respiratory tract infection, a viral condition, such as chicken pox, or influenza. The cause is unknown but the administration of aspirin may play a part. It is characterised by severe persistent vomiting and fever, followed by wild behaviour, delirium and convulsions which cause death in about 23% of sufferers. 50% have persistent mental or neurological disturbances.
>
> It occurs worldwide but is rare in western Europe. The younger the patient the higher the death rate.

rheumatic fever – an acute febrile illness which can cause arthralgia, chorea, carditis and a rash. It occurs following a strepococcal infection. The long term consequences involve damage to heart valves, deforming arthritis or neurological problems. The condition, particularly its sequelae, is less common since the advent of antibiotics.

rheumatism – a general term for painful disabling conditions affecting the joints, muscles and surrounding structures.

rheumatoid arthritis – a chronic inflammatory disease affecting the synovial lining of several joints, tendon sheaths and bursae. It is an auto-immune disease which runs a prolonged course with exacerbations and remissions and accompanied by a generalised systemic disturbance. It is approximately three times more common in women than men.

rhinitis – inflammation of the mucous membrane lining the nose.

rhinophyma – an enlargement of the nose due to the enormous enlargement of sebaceous glands sometimes occurring in the later stages of rosacea.

rhinoplasty – a repair of the nose by an operation; normally carried out by a plastic or an ear, nose and throat surgeon. Sometimes referred to as a 'nose job' if carried out for purely cosmetic reasons but the operation may be surgically necessary following injury.

rhizotomy – an operation to cut a nerve root to relieve pain.

rhonchi – harsh sound, like snoring or whistling heard over the bronchial tubes often during infection or during an attack of asthma.

rickets – a deficiency disease occurring in children due to a shortage of vitamin D or insufficient exposure to sunlight, which creates vitamin D from substances in the skin. It is characterised by a loss of appetite, vomiting and diarrhoea with clay coloured stools, convulsions and tenderness of the bones with a delay in learning to sit up. It goes on to cause distortion, softening and bending of incompletely mineralised bones some times producing nodules over the ribs. 'Renal rickets' is not a deficiency disease but a congenital inability of the kidneys to reabsorb phosphates necessary for normal bone structure.

Rift Valley fever – a virus disease transmitted by mosquitos, at one time confined to sub Sahara Africa, predominantly occurring in domestic animals like cattle, sheep and goats. In man it causes fever, haemorrhages, encephalitis with involvement of the eye. In 1977 the disease flared up in Egypt as a human infection and is now threatening the whole Middle East.

rigidity – a term used in neurology meaning stiffness and resistance to movement. Smooth rigidity is known as spastic, while jerky rigidity is known as cogwheel. The latter is a sign of Parkinsonism.

rigor – another name for shivering.

ringworm – an inflammatory infection of the skin produced by the fungus Tinea, such as Tinea capitis (the head), cruris (the groin), pedis (the feet) unguinium (the nails) etc.

risus sardonicus – the facial appearance when the muscles of the forehead go into spasm in tetanus, giving the effect of a sardonic grin.

Rocky Mountain spotted fever – a fever of the typhus group caused by Rickettsia rickettsii. It was first reported in the Rocky Mountain states of the U.S.A, but can be found in all parts of that country.

rodent ulcer – a chronic form of ulcer about the nose and face of elderly people. It is also referred to as a basal cell carcinoma as it is a malignant growth occurring in the basal cells of the skin.

rombergism – an unsteadiness on standing with the eyes shut. It is a sign in some nervous diseases such as peripheral neuropathy and tabes dorsalis. It has been referred to as 'the wash basin syndrome' because of the tendency to fall forwards into the wash basin before the eyes are fully open in the morning!

rosacea – another name for acne rosacea, a condition characterised by chronic congestion and flushing of the face and forehead with the formation of red papules. At first it waxes and wanes after meals and alcohol excess, but ultimately it becomes permanent with gross enlargement of the sebaceous glands and rhinophyma (qv).

rosiola – any rose coloured rash.

Rous sarcoma – a malignant tumour of fowls due to a virus. The tumour is the subject of experimental work upon the nature of cancer.

Royal Free disease – see neuromyaesthenia.

rubella – another name for German measles.

rupture – another name for hernia.

sacroileitis – inflammation of one or both the sacroiliac joints (between the sacrum and the ileum). It may result from ankylosing spondylitis, Reiter's syndrome or the arthritis associated with psoriasis.

sadism – a form of sexual perversion where satisfaction is derived from inflicting cruelty (after the Marquis de Sade).

St. Vitus Dance – the former name for chorea.

salmonellosis – food poisoning due to salmonella organisms.

salmon patches – pink patches found in some newborn infants on the eyelids, between the eyes and the nape of the neck. In the first two places they have usually faded by the first birthday while those on the nape of the neck are most persistent.

salpingitis – inflammation of or in the fallopian tubes.

sandfly fever – a short sharp fever occurring in parts of the tropics and sub-tropics due to a virus conveyed by a small hairy midge or sandfly.

> **salicylism** – a condition produced by an overdose of drugs of the aspirin family and characterised by ringing in the ears, rapid breathing, nausea, visual disturbances and dizziness.

sarcoidosis – a chronic disease involving the skin, lymph nodes, salivary glands, the lungs, heart, hands and feet. The condition somewhat resembles tuberculosis.

scabies – a skin disease caused by the mite, Sarcopti scabei. The female burrows into the skin particularly in front of the wrists, the web and side of the fingers, buttocks, genitalia and feet. The mite lays her eggs and the lateral movement of the larvae causes intense itching giving scabies the popular name of 'itch'. It is rife in Great Britain.

scanning speech – a speech disorder whereby syllables are articulated wrongly in a short form and each given the same vocal emphasis. It is a result of disease of the cerebellum or its connecting nerves.

scar – the result of a healed wound, ulcer or breach of tissue. It is made up of fibrous tissue.

scarlet fever – an infectious disease caused by the erythrogenic toxin of the streptococcus. It is characterised by fever, headache, vomiting and a punctate erythematous rash following a streptococcal infection of the throat. The skin subsequently peels. In the latter part of the 19th century it was the commonest cause of death in children or infants which had decreased by 1900 and ceased by 1965.

schistosomiasis – a parasitic disease of the tropics acquired by wading in fresh water where forms of the blood fluke penetrate the skin and migrate to various organs via the bloodstream. The reservoirs of the disease are snails in which the eggs of the parasite develop into larvae. The disease is also known as bilharzia.

schizophrenia – a collective name given to a group of conditions characterised, during an acute episode, by hallucinations (e.g. voices), strange experiences (e.g. mental and bodily functions being interfered with by outside forces) and the inability to think clearly, along with bizarre speech and behaviour. Previously known as dementia praecox.

> 'The wounded surgeon plies the steel,
> That questions the distempered part;
> Beneath the bleeding hands we feel
> The sharp compassion of the healer's art
> Resolving the enigma of the fever chart'.
>
> From East Coker
> *(T.S. Eliot 1888-1965)*

sciatica – pain in the path of distribution of the sciatic nerve. It occurs in the buttocks going on to the back of the thigh, the outside and front of the leg.

scirrus – a hard form of cancer made up mostly of fibrous tissue.

scleritis – a disease of the eye due to inflammation of the sclera.

scleroderma – a condition in which the skin becomes hard, like leather, causing stiffening of the joints and gradual wasting of the muscles. It has the appearance of the skin being too tight to cover the body. It is a disease of connective tissue of unknown cause. The condition can progress to affect the lungs, heart, digestive tract and kidneys.

sclerosis – a hardening of tissue, especially by overgrowth of fibrous tissue. It affects many kinds of tissue e.g. nerve tissue (multiple sclerosis), and the linings of the arteries (arteriosclerosis).

scoliosis – an abnormal curvature of the spine which bends to one side and is rotated laterally.

scotoma – an area of blindness in the field of vision.

scrivener's palsy – writer's cramp.

scrofula – tuberculosis glands of the neck. The condition was also known as King's Evil to be cured by the royal touch, dating from Edward the Confessor.

scrombotoxin poisoning – caused by eating poorly preserved scrombal fish e.g. tuna, mackerel and other fish of the mackerel family, which produce a toxin of a histamine-like substance. The symptoms include nausea, vomiting headaches, upper abdominal pain, urticaria and itching.

scrum pox – a contagious infection affecting forward rugby players as a result of face to face contact. It may take the form of impetigo or herpes simplex. It is sometimes referred to as 'prop pox' (although one must assume that hookers aren't exempt!).

scurvy – a deficiency disease due to lack of vitamin C and characterised by the extravasation of the blood into the tissues of the body. Advanced scurvy, which is now rare, gives rise to spongy bleeding gums, loose teeth and haemorrhages under the skin. Mild scurvy due to food aversion, poor diet or inadequate food supplements of infant foods still occurs occasionally.

LIMEYS & POMS?

Scurvy is a disease which has existed wherever people are forced to live without fresh fruit and vegetables.

Although, historically, it is usually associated with long sea voyages, it was rife among the French army in the Crimea and it attacked both sides in the American civil war.

A Scottish naval surgeon, James Lind, discovered that fresh fruit or lemon juice could prevent and cure the disease. Lind published his findings in 1753 as 'A Treatise on the Scurvy'.

This discovery was to benefit the crews of Captain James Cook on their voyage to the South Pacific. Because English seamen were supplied with lime juice on their voyages they became referred to as 'limeys', a soubriquet which has been extended to Englishmen in general, most commonly used by Americans.

sea sickness – a characteristic set of symptoms experienced by many people due to the rolling or rocking of a vessel at sea (see motion sickness).

seat worm – another name for thread worm.

sebaceous cyst – a cyst in the skin found as a result of the blockage of a duct of a sebaceous gland.

seborrhoea – a group of diseases in which sebaceous oil-forming glands are at fault. It causes an accumulation of dry scurf or the formation of excessive oily deposits on otherwise healthy skin. Seborrhoeic dermatitis is another name for eczema.

self poisoning – one of the commonest causes of admission to hospital and is due to the self ingestion of poisonous agents such as drugs.

sepsis – poisoning by the products of the growth of micro–organisms. In the body the general symptoms are those of inflammation.

septicaemia – multiplication of bacteria in the blood (see blood poisoning).

sequelae – the symptoms or effects following certain diseases.

serpiginous – a term used in connection with ulcers or eruptions which spread in a creepy manner.

serum sickness – a hypersensitivity reaction due to circulating antigen/antibody complexes. It is the reaction to the administration of foreign serum given as a form of passive immunisation before the days of antibiotics. It is characterised by fever, arthralgia and lymphadenopathy and is self-limiting.

shaking palsy – another name for Parkinsonism.

> **shellfish poisoning** – may be a cause of typhoid fever or paralytic shellfish poisoning which is caused by a toxin that accumulates in mussels, cockles and scallops. This form is characterised by a loss of feeling in the limbs, tingling in the tongue and difficulty in breathing.

shell shock – a form of war neurosis which presented a major medical problem in the 1914-1918 war.

shingles – see zoster.

shock – the state of acute circulatory failure in which cardiac output is inadequate to provide normal perfusion of the body's organs. It is a failure of flow rate rather than a failure of blood pressure. It is characterised by a lowered blood pressure.

short sight – objects near at hand are seen clearly but those at a distance appear blurred. Another name for the condition is myopia.

> **sickle cell anaemia** – a form of anaemia in black people because of the sickle shape of the red blood cells. It is caused by the presence of abnormal haemoglobin which makes the blood cells more fragile. This is responsible for the anaemia.

siderosis – a chronic fibrosis of the lung in iron workers due to inhalation of particles. There can also be deposits of iron in the tissues of the body.

silicosis – a form of pneumoconiosis caused by the inhalation of free silica. It occurs in pottery workers, coal miners, sand blasters, tin miners and metal grinders.

Simmond's disease – a condition occurring as a result of the destruction of the pituitary gland, characterised by wasting of the skin, the bones, impotence, loss of hair, low basal metabolic rate and low blood pressure. One cause is post-partum necrosis of the gland following severe interpartum or post-partum haemorrhage; sometimes referred to as pituitary cachexia.

singer's nodule – a small swelling on the vocal cords causing hoarseness which tends to develop in people who abuse their voices.

singulitis – the Latin name for hiccup.

sinusitis – inflammation of the sinuses of the face. It can occur following a cold or upper respiratory tract infection if the drainage channels of the sinuses become blocked.

> **Sjörgren's syndrome** – a condition characterised by dryness of the mouth and eye associated with rheumatoid arthritis. It occurs in about 10% of patients with rheumatoid arthritis but can occur independently of the disease. A specific HLA antigen is mostly present in sufferers.

slapped cheek disease – erythema of the face.

sleeping sickness (African trypanosomiasis) – a condition which occurs in West, East and Central Africa between 14°N and 25°S latitude. The condition is characterised by lethargy and a constant tendency to sleep which can proceed to emaciation and death. It is due to the parasites Trypanosoma gambiense in man while other forms of the parasite only affect cattle. The parasite is transmitted by the tse tse fly.

sleepy sickness – a popular name for encephalitis lethargica, a virus infection of the brain.

slipped disc – another name for prolapsed intervertebral disc.

small pox – the condition was so called to distinguish it from syphilis (the great pox). Until recently small pox was one of the major killing diseases. It was a highly infectious viral disease sometimes called variola. The disease has been eradicated by mass vaccination programmes. The last naturally occurring case was reported in October 1977 and on May 8th 1980 the World Health Organisation declared the disease eradicated.

EDWARD JENNER (1749-1823), was a country physician practising in Gloucestershire when he became interested in the disease cowpox, which affected the hands of milkmaids and others handling the teats and udders of infected cows. He became aware that those affected did not appear to catch the more serious disease, small pox.

In 1796 Jenner took some matter from the pustules on the affected hands of a milkmaid, Sarah Nelmes and used it to vaccinate an 8 year old boy, James Phipps. He then inoculated the boy with small pox. The boy did not contract the disease.

The practise of vaccination met with violent opposition from some of the medical establishment. However, eventually 70 prominent physicians and surgeons in London signed a declaration of confidence in the process. It then became acceptable.

snake bite – poisoning resulting from the bite of a snake usually of the viper or cobra family. It is characterised by swelling and paralysis of the bitten part followed by palpitations and difficulty in breathing.

snow blindness – is caused by exposure to ultra violet light reflected from the snow fields giving rise to pain and watering of the eyes and photophobia. Treatment is to keep the eye covered for 24 hours.

soft sore (chancroid) – venereal ulceration due to haemophilus ducreyi which is common in the tropics and sub–tropics.

soldiers heart – see effort syndrome.

somnambulism – sleep walking.

sore – a popular name for an ulcer.

spasm – means involuntary and in some cases, painful contraction of a muscle or of a hollow organ with a muscular wall.

spasmodic torticollis – a chronic condition in which the neck is rotated or deviated laterally, forwards or backwards with additional jerking or tremor.

spasmophilia – a condition affecting certain people especially in childhood in which motor nerves are usually sensitive to irritation. There is also an abnormal tendency to convulsions, while spasms only can occur in very slight cases.

spasmus notans – rhythmic nodding of the head.

spastic – a condition where there is increased muscular tone. A spastic gait is associated with some diseases of the upper part of the nervous system (upper neurone).

spermatorrhoea – the passage of semen without erection of the penis or orgasm.

spina bifida – a congenital malformation of the spine in which some of the vertebrae fail to fuse so that a sac containing the covers of the spinal cord and even the spinal cord itself protrude under the skin. The condition is present at birth and it may result in paralysis and incontinence and may also be associated with hydrocephalus.

spinner's finger – a cricket injury. Bowlers are liable to get callosities of the finger of the bowling hand which tend to crack.

splenectomy – operation for the removal of the spleen.

splenic anaemia – enlargement of the spleen associated with anaemia. It is also known as Banti's disease.

splenomegaly – enlargement of the spleen.

splinter haemorrhages – linear bleeding under the finger nail which may result from injury but is also a useful sign of infective endocarditis.

spondylitis – see ankylosing spondylitis.

spondylolisthesis – a congenital defect of the spine usually affecting the fifth lumbar vertebra. There is a slipping forward of the affected vertebra.

spondylosis – a degenerative lesion of the spine leading to ankylosis.

spondylosis (cervical) – is a spondylosis affecting the vertebrae of the neck

spotted fever – an epidemic form of cerebrospinal fever. It also refers to meningitis and typhus.

sprains – injury in the neighbourhood of joints usually with tearing of the ligaments and effusion of blood.

> **sprue** – a chronic, usually tropical disease, characterised by diarrhoea, emaciation and anaemia due to deficient absorption of food from the small intestine (see malabsorption syndrome).

squint – the visual axis of each eye are not directed simultaneously at the same fixed point. Squints can be convergent or divergent. The more correct term is strabismus.

stammering – a disruption of the normal flow of speech. There is an intrusion of pauses and repetitions especially of initial consonants into one's speaking either due to a speech disorder or through tension or fear.

stannosis – a form of pneumoconiosis caused by the inhalation of stannic oxide in those mining tin ore.

stasis – a stoppage of the flow of blood in the vessels or of food materials down the intestinal canal.

steathorrhoea – the passage of stools containing fat.

stenosis – an unnatural narrowing of any passage or orifice of the body. It is of particular importance in the four openings in the heart and in the intestinal tract.

steppage gait – a peculiar walk characteristic of neuritis affecting the muscles of the legs causing drop foot. The feet are lifted high so that the toes may clear the ground.

stertor – a term applied to noisy breathing.

Stevens-Johnson syndrome – a form of erythema characterised by annular lesions which can develop into blisters. There can be involvement of the eyes and mucosa giving rise to ulceration. It is most commonly due to a hypersensitivity reaction to certain drugs particularly the sulphonamides and has a 25% mortality rate.

staghorn calculus – a large stone which more or less fills the pelvis of the kidney and has irregular projecting surfaces resembling antlers.

> **Stein-Leventhal syndrome** – a rare condition characterised by sterility, absence of menstruation and hirsutism in women having enlarged ovaries with many cysts. Treatment is the surgical removal of a wedge-shaped section of the tissue from each ovary.

sthenic – a term applied to certain diseases indicating that they are not associated with prostration.

stigma – a spot or impression on the skin.

Still's disease – juvenile rheumatoid arthritis described by Sir Frederic Still (1868-1911). The arthritis is usually symmetrical and starts in the fingers which become spindle shaped. There is often marked wasting due to the child not wanting to move the painful joints. The onset is usually between 2 and 5 and is self-limiting but there is a tendency to relapse and it may persist for years.

stitch – a popular name for a sharp pain in the side generally due to cramp following unusually hard exertion. It should not be confused with pleurisy or fractured ribs.

Stokes-Adams syndrome – a condition in which the slowness of the pulse is associated with attacks of unconsciousness due to a state of heart block. Nowadays it can be alleviated by the use of a pacemaker.

> ROBERT ADAMS (1791-1875) was a Dublin physician noted for his contribution to the knowledge of heart disease and gout. He described the condition of slow pulse and giddiness proceeding to convulsive seizures which became known as Stokes Adams attacks, after himself and another Dublin physician William Stokes (1804-1878), who also described this condition.

stoma – an opening constructed when the bowel has to be brought to the skin surface to convey gastrointestinal or bladder contents. It comes from the Greek word meaning mouth. There are three principle types of stoma: a colostomy (100,000 in U.K.), ileostomy (10,000) and urostomy (2,000).

stomatitis – inflammation of the mouth.

strabismus – see squint.

strangury – a condition in which there is a constant desire to pass urine accompanied by a straining sensation with only a few drops voided. It is associated with inflammation in the kidney, bladder and urinary passages.

stress fracture – a type of fracture common in sportsmen and women following an undue amount of exercise, an amount he or she is not capable of coping with in his or her state of training. There is pain over the affected bone which is insidious in onset and worse at night and during and after exercise.

striae atrophicae – a term applied to atrophied strips of skin where it has been excessively stretched. In pregnancy they are referred to as striae gravidarum.

stricture – a narrowing in any of the natural passages of the body e.g. the gullet, bowel or urethra. It is usually caused by previous ulceration or some growth in the wall or pressure from a growth in a neighbouring organ.

stridor – a noise associated with inspiration due to a narrowing of the upper airway, particularly the larynx.

stroke – sudden insensibility or body disablement connected with some disease condition of the brain, which is sometimes referred to as a cerebrovascular accident or apoplexy. It can be caused by a clot in a blood vessel of the brain, a cerebral embolus, disease in the vessel wall, cerebral thrombosis, or, more serious, a cerebral haemorrhage. The symptoms may vary but the sequelae may give rise to a serious form of disablement such as hemiplegia or loss of the power of speech.

strongyloidosis – infestation with the nematode strongylus which occurs in the tropics, particularly in the Far East. It gives rise to an itching skin rash, creeping eruption, severe diarrhoea, severe anaemia and prostration.

strophulus – also known as red gum. The condition produces a rash of red pimples in young children about teething time. It is caused by excess sweating.

struma – an old term applied to a swelling of the neck due either to a tuberculous gland or an enlarged thyroid. It therefore referred to either scrofula or goitre.

strychnine poisoning – the condition quickly causes convulsions. There are brief flaccid periods between the convulsions. The mental faculties are unaffected and the condition ends in death or recovery within a short time. The convulsions bear some resemblance to the spasms of tetanus.

stye – a suppurative inflammation of one of the glands at the margin of the eyelid.

sub-acute combined degeneration of the cord – a degenerative condition of the spinal cord which most commonly occurs as a complication of pernicious anaemia. It is characterised by sensory loss in the limbs (glove and stocking) along with motor symptoms especially in the lower limbs.

subacute sclerosing panencephalitis – a rare complication of measles due to infection of the brain by the measles virus. It can occur 2-18 years after the onset of measles causing mental deterioration leading to coma or death. The condition occurs in 1.1 million children and it is 5-20 times greater in incidence following the disease than following the vaccine.

subarachnoid haemorrhage – haemorrhage into the subarachnoid space of the brain usually as a result of the rupture of an aneurysm in one of the blood vessels making up the 'circle of Willis'.

THOMAS WILLIS (1621-1675) was an English physician and one of the founders of the Royal Society (1662). He became famous as a physician at Westminster and was a pioneer in the study of the anatomy of the brain and diseases of the nervous system and muscles. He discovered the arrangement of blood vessels, known as the circle of Willis, in a part of the brain. In 1664 he wrote 'Cerebri Anatomi'.

subinvolution – the womb fails to undergo the usual decrease in size after child birth.

subluxation – a partial dislocation.

sudàmina – a small vesicle appearing under the surface area of the skin during diseases associated with constant perspiration.

sudden infant death syndrome – another name for cot death.

suffocation – asphyxia or choking.

suicide – an act or an instance of intentionally killing oneself.

sulphaemoglobin – an abnormal pigment found in the blood as the result of interaction between certain drugs derived from aniline.

sunburn – inflammation or blistering of the skin due to over exposure to direct sunlight or a sunlamp.

superfoetation – fertilisation of a second ovum in a woman already pregnant.

superinvolution – the womb decreases in size after childbirth to such an extent that there is more or less complete wasting of the organ.

suppuration – the process of pus formation.

swimmer's ear – a fungus infection of the ear canal similar to athlete's foot.

sycosis – a skin disease in which the hair follicles, especially of the chin, are inflamed forming pustules around the hair and the surrounding area of the skin becomes swollen and reddened; the infection is usually due to a staphylococcus or ringworm.

Sydenham's chorea – see chorea.

sympathetic disease – a disease or symptoms in one part arising as a consequence of disease in a distant part.

sympathetic ophthalmia – inflammation of one eye due to injury to the other eye. Prompt treatment of an injured eye is important to prevent involvement of the other eye and possible blindness.

syncope – another name for fainting, a loss of consciousness due to a fall of blood pressure.

syndactyly – webbed or fused fingers or toes.

synechiae – an adhesion between the iris and adjacent structures (the cornea and iris) arising as a result of inflammation of the iris.

synganosis – a disease of the lungs caused by roundworm Synganus laryngeii. Occurs in the Caribbean and is characterised by a persistent cough, fever, haemoptysis and loss of weight. Sometimes the patient coughs up the red wriggly worms. If not, the worms can be removed through a bronchoscope.

synostosis – the uniting of the bony material from adjacent bones normally separate.

synovitis– inflammation of the membrane lining the joint. This may be due to a number of causes such as acute rheumatism, injuries, inflammation of the joints and, in a chronic form, tuberculosis.

syphilis – a chronic infectious and contagious venereal disease caused by the spirochaete, Treponema pallidum and usually transmitted during sexual intercourse. It also passes from mother to foetus during pregnancy. It progresses through three stages characterised by the local formation of a chancre (primary syphilis), ulcerous skin eruptions or a brief transient rash (secondary syphilis) and systemic infection leading to numerous possible conditions affecting different systems of the body (tertiary syphilis). The latter include gummata (skin), diseased heart valves and aneurysms (cardiovascular system) and tabes dorsalis and general paralysis of the insane (central nervous system).

syringomyelia – a chronic disease of the central nervous system involving the spinal cord with the presence of fluid filled cavities in the cord leading to spasticity and loss of awareness of pain and temperature. If there is involvement of the brain it is called syringobulbia.

T

tabes – the term literally means wasting, but it usually refers to tabes dorsalis or locomotor ataxia, one of the consequences of tertiary syphilis. The lesions are in the posterior horns of the spinal cord. The patient demonstrates a loss of sensation in the limbs with disorganised joints and characteristic pupil changes.

tache cerebral – a bright red line of congestion when a finger is drawn across the patient's skin in meningitis.

tachycardia – rapid pulse rate.

tachypnoea – unusual quickness of breathing.

taenia – infestation due to the taenia or tapeworm species caused by the consumption of under-cooked beef, fish or pork.

Tay-Sachs disease – an hereditary disease occurring mostly in Jewish children manifested in early infancy by weakness in the muscles and blindness. A bright cherry spot is present at the back of the eye. There is no treatment and life expectancy is short.

teeth grinding – see bruxism.

teichopsia – zig zag lines which patients with migraine often see.

telangiectasis – dilatation of groups of small blood vessels appearing as fine red or blue lines on the skin, sometimes associated with diseases of the skin, cirrhosis of the liver and other disorders.

tendovaginitis – inflammation of a tendon and the sheath enveloping it.

tenesmus – painful straining to empty the bowel but without success. It is a symptom of diseases affecting the large intestine such as dysentery, piles or tumours.

tennis elbow – tenosynovitis around the elbow.

tenosynovitis – inflammation of a tendon.

tenotomy – operation to divide one or more tendons, usually to remedy a deformity.

teratogenesis – the production of physical defects in the foetus during development. It can be the result of inappropriate drug administration during pregnancy e.g. thalidomide.

tertian fever – applied to a type of malaria in which fever occurs every other day.

tetanus – a serious infection caused by the toxins produced by the bacterial organism, Clostridium tetani. The organisms enter the body through perforating, penetrating or deep wounds. They thrive in the absence of oxygen. The main manifestations are violent spasms of the muscles. The disease is easily preventable by the administration of tetanus toxoid immunisation. The condition is also known as lockjaw.

tetany – spasm of muscles caused by the fall in ionic calcium in the blood. The condition can be due to hypoparathyroidism. A sign to elucidate the spasms is Chvostek's sign which consists of tapping the facial muscle and causing it to go into spasms.

tetralogy of Fallot – the commonest form of cyanotic congenital heart disease. The tetralogy consists of: stenosis of the pulmonary valve, ventricular septal defect, overriding aorta and right ventricular hypertrophy.

thalassaemia – see Cooley's anaemia.

thoracocentesis – withdrawal of fluid from the pleural cavity.

thoracoplasty – the removal of a varying number of ribs so that the underlying lung collapses. The operation was carried out to rest that part of the lung in tuberculosis.

thrill – a vibration or tremor felt on applying the hand to the surface of the body over the heart in conditions with a narrowing of the valve opening.

thromboangitis obliterans – another name for Buerger's disease.

thrombocytopenia – the absence or diminution of platelets or thrombocytes in the blood. These are necessary for blood coagulation so the condition results in bleeding from tiny blood vessels into the skin and mucous membranes (see purpura).

thrombophlebitis – inflammation of the veins with clot formation. The veins of the leg are most commonly affected and if superficial the affected vein may be felt as a tender cord.

thrombosis – the formation of a blood clot within blood vessels or in the heart lining. The most familiar example is coronary thrombosis but many other vessels other than those supplying the heart can be involved.

> **thrower's fracture** – a fracture of the humerus caused by the muscular force generated in a hard throw.

thrush – a type of inflammation affecting particularly the mouth of weakly children causing white patches to appear on the lips, tongue or palate, caused by the growth of a fungus on the surface of the mucous membranes, usually candida. Vaginal thrush is the name given to candidiasis of the vagina.

thyrotoxic adenoma – a variety of thyrotoxicosis in which one of the nodules of a multinodular goitre becomes autonomous and secretes excess thyroid hormone producing a similar condition to thyrotoxicosis.

thyrotoxicosis – see Graves' disease.

tic – term applied to habit spasm which forms a personal peculiarity in neurotic subjects.

tic douloureux – another name for facial or trigeminal neuralgia due to some affection of the fifth cranial nerve and characterised by pain situated somewhere about the temple, forehead face and jaw sometimes with spasms of the affected region.

tinea – another name for ringworm.

tinea cruris – ringworm of the groin; a fungus infection of the skin of the upper thighs near the genital organs (Dhobi itch).

tinnitus – a noise heard in the ear without any external cause. It frequently accompanies deafness.

tired arm syndrome – aching and throbbing pain in the upper limbs sometimes with weakness, occurring at night, mainly in middle aged women.

titubation – staggery or reeling. A condition especially due to disease of the spinal cord or cerebellum.

> **tonsillitis** – inflammation of the tonsils; the condition is never entirely confined to the tonsils and there is always some involvement of the surrounding throat or pharynx. Tonsillitis is usually caused by a beta haemolytic streptococcus but it may occur in infectious mononucleosis and is also associated with diphtheria.

tophus – a concretion formed in connection with joints or tendon sheaths as a result of an attack of gout.

tormina – a technical name for griping pain felt around the naval as a result of spasmodic action of the muscle coat in the small intestine. (colic).

torpor – a condition of bodily or mental inactivity not amounting to sleep but interfering greatly with ordinary habits. It occurs in those suffering from fever and in elderly people with diseased arteries.

torsion – a twisting process in which organs or tumours attached by pedicles become twisted and constrict the blood supply e.g. the testis.

torticollis – shortness of the sternomastoid muscle on one side resulting in asymmetry and limitation of movement.

toxaemia – a form of blood poisoning due to absorption of bacterial products (toxins) formed at some local site of infection such as an abscess. In some cases the term toxaemia can refer to defective action in some excretory organs such as the kidney.

Toxaemia of pregnancy indicates pre-eclampsia (high blood pressure, albuminuria and oedema) or full blown eclampsia.

> **toxic shock syndrome** – first described in 1978 and characterised by high fever, diarrhoea, shock and an erythematous rash. The condition can be due to tampons, but it has been described in men. The cause is the staphylococcus toxin. It has a 10% mortality rate.

toxocariasis – a disease acquired by swallowing the ova of a roundworm which lives in the intestine of cats (Toxocara cati) or dogs (Toxocara canis) . The larvae migrate to various parts of the body including the retina where they die and produce small granulomata. These produce an allergic reaction and, in the eye, may cause choroid-retinitis.

toxoplasmosis – a disease caused by infection with a microorganism, Toxoplasma gondii, which usually produces only mild symptoms except if contracted by a pregnant woman when it can give rise to blindness and mental retardation in the foetus.

tracheitis – inflammation of the trachea; it may occur on its own or in association with bronchitis or laryngitis.

tracheostomy – an operation on the wind pipe which is opened from the front of the neck and which allows air to enter directly into air passages. The operation may be carried out in an emergency.

trachoma – a disease of the eye characterised by inflammation and scarring. It is caused by the organism Chlamydia trachomatis and is the leading preventable cause of blindness worldwide. It occurs in the tropics and is only found in the U.K. in the immigrant population. It can be treated by tetracyclines.

trance – a profound sleep from which a person cannot be brought round. It is not due to any organic disease but can be due to hysteria or induced by hypnosis.

transient ischaemic attacks – consists of episodes of transient ischaemia in some parts of the cerebral hemisphere or the brain stem and lasts for a few minutes to several hours. It is due to atheroma of the carotid or vertebral arteries due to emboli or cholesterol. It presents as a stroke which rapidly gets better.

trans-sexualism – a psycho-sexual abnormality characterised by a feeling of belonging to the opposite gender to those of their genitalia and secondary sex characteristics.

transvestism – a psycho-sexual abnormality with a repetitive compulsion to dress in clothes of the opposite sex to achieve orgasm.

trauma – a term used to indicate disorders due to a wound or injury.

travellers' diarrhoea – an infection, usually due to Escherichia coli, associated with fever, diarrhoea and vomiting; also known as Basra belly, Delhi belly, gippy tummy, Montezuma's revenge etc. etc.

travel sickness – sickness induced by any form of transport.

tremor – a fine kind of involuntary movement involving the projecting parts such as the hands, fingers and tongue.

trench fever – an infectious disease caused by the organism Rickettsia quintana transmitted by the body louse. There were large epidemics in the 1914–1918 war.

trench foot – see immersion foot.

trench mouth – see Vincent's angina.

treponema – a genus of spirochaetal organisms. Treponema pallidum is the cause of syphilis.

trichiasis – the eyelashes become ingrown.

> **trichinosis** – a disease due to eating diseased pork infested with Trichinella spirosis. It is characterised by intestinal disorders, fever, muscular swelling, pain and delirium.

trichomonas vaginalis – a protozoa normally present in the vagina of 30-40% of women, which sometimes becomes pathogenic causing inflammation and a greenish vaginal discharge. It may infect men giving rise to a urethral discharge. It is necessary to treat both partners.

trichorrhoea – a term applied to the falling out of the hair usually due to some general condition e.g. scarlet fever or typhoid.

> **trichotillomania** – a condition in which a person has an obsessive impulse to pull out his own hair.

trichuriasis – worldwide infection common in tropics and caused by Trichuris trichuria or whip worm. The condition is due to eating vegetables and drinking infected water polluted by the eggs of the worm. The worms seldom cause trouble but in under-nourished children they may cause bleeding from the bowels.

trigeminal neuralgia – see tic douloureux.

trigger finger – a condition in which efforts to unbend a finger are at first unsuccessful but it can soon straighten with a snap or a jerk. It is caused by a constriction preventing free movement of a tendon in its sheath.

trismus – another name for lockjaw.

trypanosomiasis – sleeping sickness.

tsutsugimushi – Japanese river fever, a disease of the typhus group.

tuberculide – any skin lesion resulting from infection with the TB bacillus.

tuberculosis – general name for a whole group of diseases associated with the organism Mycobacterium tuberculi and manifesting itself in diseases of the lung, bone and other parts of the body.

ROBERT KOCH (1843 - 1910) was a German physician and pioneer bacteriologist. In 1882 he discovered the tubercle bacillus (sometimes referred to as Koch's bacillus) and in 1883 he identified the cholera organism as a result of a German expedition to Egypt in a quest for the discovery of the cholera germ.

He became the first director of the Berlin Institute for infectious diseases in 1891 and in 1905 was awarded the Nobel prize for physiology and medicine.

tuberose sclerosis – an hereditary disease due to a developmental abnormality of the brain. It gives rise to mental retardation and epilepsy, starting before the age of 2. Small nodules or tumours develop on the face as well (epiloia).

tularaemia – an infectious disease caused by the bacterium Francisella tularensis transmitted by infected rodents to humans by flies or by handling infected animals. It is characterised by fever and swelling of the lymph nodes.

tumour – a swelling.

tunnel worm – another name for ancylostoma.

Turner's syndrome – hypogonadism and infertility due to the presence of an X instead of an XX set of chromosomes in the female. It is associated with retardation of growth, failure of pubertal development, congenital cardiac abnormalities and webbing of the neck.

tympanites – distension of the abdomen due to the presence of air and gas in the abdominal cavity. On percussion the abdomen produces a noise like a note on a percussion instrument.

typhoid – an infectious fever characterised by an ulceration of the small intestine, with a rose-coloured eruption and enlargement of the spleen, caused by the typhoid bacillus.

Apart from contaminated water and food, typhoid can be spread by carriers of the organism through handling food. The most famous carrier was Mary Mallon, a cook in the early 20th century. She was known to have infected 53 people (5 fatal) and was suspected of initiating an outbreak in Ithaca, New York, in which some 1300 cases developed. Mary Mallon subsequently became known by the soubriquet 'Typhoid Mary'.

typhus – a rickettsial infection transmitted to man by infected lice and fleas from rats and mice. There are several varieties of the disease. It is endemic in parts of Asia, the near East, India and other areas.

ulcer – a break in the surface of the skin or surface of a membranous lining of any cavity within the body.

ulcerative colitis – inflammation of the colon and rectum characterised by ulcers inside the lumen on the intestinal wall and associated with bloody diarrhoea. The condition may be mild and respond readily to medical treatment or so severe as to require the surgical removal of the affected part or whole of the colon.

ulitis – inflammation of the gums.

uncinaria – another name for hookworm (ancylostoma).

uncinate fit – a type of fit where the sufferer has hallucinations of smell or taste.

unconsciousness – a condition depending usually on some disorder of the brain.

TAKE CARE

Have you noticed how inquisitive children are? You were (presumably) a child yourself at one time. Never leave, within the reach of children, bottles containing corrosive liquid. Place them in a cupboard above their reach.

You'll sleep much more soundly.

undulant fever – another name for brucellosis.

uraemia – a clinical state arising from renal failure which is caused by disease of the kidney or pre-renal causes due to a lack of circulating blood volume inadequately perfusing the organ. In uraemia there is excess urea in the blood producing acute symptoms within a few days whereas chronic uraemia occurs over a long period; the symptoms are headache in the front or back of the head, insomnia at night and drowsiness during the day, leading to deep unconsciousness, sometimes convulsions like epilepsy, vomiting and poor appetite. Diarrhoea is a serious sign.

uranorrhaphy – the operation for closure of a cleft palate.

urethritis – inflammation of the urethra characterised by cystitis-like pain and interference with the passage of urine due to a stricture or narrowing of the urethral tube. The condition can be due to non-specific urethritis, gonorrhoea, the passage of a stone, catheterisation or drugs and diet e.g. alcohol.

urethral stricture – an abrupt narrowing at one or more places in the urethra.

urticaria – an eruption on the skin, which may be general or localised, usually lasting only a few hours. It may be due to internal or external causes (sting of insects or nettle; eating of shellfish). Also known as nettle rash.

uricaemia – excessive amounts of uric acid in the blood.

uveitis – inflammation of the uveal tract or middle coat of the eye which includes the iris, ciliary body and choroid. The condition is associated with a number of general diseases such as arthritis, tuberculosis, syphilis, bowel diseases, virus diseases and diseases due to parasites and fungi.

vaccinia – another name for cow pox which presents as vesicles on the animals' teats and udders. It is caused by the same virus as smallpox and rendered those infected immune from the latter.

vaginismus – spasmodic contraction of the orifice of the vagina on attempting intercourse. It is usually psychologically caused due to a neurotic temperament or frigidity but it may be due to some local inflammatory condition.

vaginitis – inflammation of the vagina.

vagotomy – the operation of cutting fibres of the vagus nerve to the stomach which is sometimes a part of the surgical treatment of duodenal ulcers to reduce the flow of acid to the stomach.

valgus – outward displacement from the body leading to knock knees or flat feet when affecting the ankles.

varicella – another name for chicken pox.

varicocoele – a condition in which the veins of the testicle are distended.

varicose ulcers – ulcers occurring in the lower limbs due to a stagnant circulation caused by long standing varicose veins. They occur most commonly just above or adjacent to the ankles.

varicose veins – veins which are stretched and dilated. They can occur in different parts of the body; at the lower end of the bowel (haemorrhoids), around the testicles (varicocoele), the great saphenous vein (in the legs) and adjacent to the oesophagus (oesophageal varices – as a result of cirrhosis of the liver). Those in the leg are usually due to incompetent valves in the saphenous vein.

variola – another name for smallpox.

varioloid – a mild type of smallpox.

varix – an enlargement of a tortuous vein.

varus – a deformity of the legs causing them to bend outwards giving rise to a condition of the hip (coxa vara) of the knee (genu varum) or the ankle (talipes varus).

vasectomy – surgical operation to render men sterile or infertile by cutting the ductus or vas deferens.

venereal disease – now referred to as sexually transmitted diseases. A general name given to contagious diseases communicated from one person to another by sexual intercourse.

venereal warts – another name for condylomata.

venesection – the withdrawal of blood by opening a vein.

verbigeration – insane repetition of meaningless words or sentences.

vernix caseosa – a greasy substance that covers and waterproofs the skin of the foetus.

verruca – a wart, especially one found on the sole of the foot.

verrucose – covered with warts.

vertigo – a sense of dizziness and a feeling of whirling around either of oneself or the environment. The condition is mostly due to a disorder of the semi-circular canals of the inner ear.

vesicle – a small sac containing fluid on the skin like a skin blister.

Vincent's angina – an ulcerative inflamed condition of the mouth and gums caused by spindle-shaped bacilli, spirilla, and characterised by its foul smell. Also known as trench mouth.

viral haemorrhagic fever – a severe virus fever similar to Marburg disease.

virilism – masculine characteristics developing in the female usually as a result of overactivity of the suprarenal glands.

visceroptosis – a falling down of the viscera especially those in the abdomen. In elderly women it often occurs in association with prolapse of the womb.

vitiligo – patchy areas of depigmented skin surrounded by areas of pigmentation. It can often occur in some auto-immune diseases such as Graves' disease and Addison's disease.

Volkmann's contracture – occurs as a result of too much pressure from a splint or bandage in the treatment of a broken arm, causing the flexor muscles of the forearm to contract, obstructing the free flow of blood in the arms. The muscles then swell and become fibrosed.

volvulus – twisting or knotting of the bowel causing intestinal obstruction and sometimes leading to gangrene of a section of bowel.

vomiting – expulsion of stomach contents through the mouth. When nothing comes up it is known as wretching. Vomiting can be a sign in many diseases although it is often a transient event of no great significance.

vulvo-vaginitis – inflammation of the vulva and vagina. The condition is more common in young girls than in adult women. It may be due to infection in the vagina or a manifestation of conditions elsewhere in the body.

von Gierke's disease – a condition due to an inborn error of metabolism giving rise to a shortage of glucose-6-phosphatase. This results in glycogen storage disease with the involvement of the heart, liver and kidneys.

von Recklinghausen's disease – a condition characterised by multiple tumours in the skin along nerve pathways. The tumours are composed mainly of fibrous tissue, are non-cancerous and tend to increase in numbers. The disorder is thought to be hereditary.

warts – growths arising from skin due to a papovirus infection. Common warts of the hands, face and feet are most frequent in children and are contagious. The sufferer can easily become reinfected. Another name for a wart is a verruca but this name usually refers to the variety found on the soles of the feet.

wasp stings – these are sometimes treated by applying lemon juice or vinegar to offset the alkaline nature of the sting. In those with a known allergy, a vaccination is available.

wasting palsy – a popular name for the disease known as progressive muscular palsy.

waterbrash – another name for pyrosis.

water cancer – another name for cancrum oris.

waterhammer pulse – the type of pulse associated with an incompetent aortic valve. It has a peculiar collapsing feel.

water on the brain – a popular name for hydrocephalus or meningitis.

> **water-spread disease** – a general name given to diseases which can spread by impure water, e.g. excess sulphates (diarrhoea), excess nitrogen (methaemoglobinaemia in infants), lack of fluoride (dental caries) etc. etc.

weals (wheals) – raised white areas of skin with reddened margins. They may be a sign of nettle rash or due to injury.

webbed fingers – also called syndactyly. It is a deformity present at birth and it runs in families.

Weil's disease – see leptospirosis.

wen – a small tumour in the skin. It is another name for a sebaceous cyst.

wet brain – a term applied to the oedematous state of the brain caused by chronic alcoholism and associated with mental failure and delusions.

wheezing – a popular name applied to various sounds produced in the chest when the bronchial tubes are narrowed, particularly in asthma and bronchitis.

whelk – a popular name applied to a weal and red protuberance on the face or nose seen in hard drinkers.

whiplash injury – a popular name for the injury sustained when the head is suddenly thrown forward and jerked backwards. It may occur in car accidents. The injury is like a sprained neck whereby the muscles and ligaments are strained and torn but rarely with damage to bones and nerves.

Whipple's disease – a rare progressive disease of unknown cause characterised by arthritis, fever, fatty stools, diarrhoea, loss of weight, lymph node enlargement, loss of strength and abnormalities of the small intestine.

whip worm – one of the most common of the worms parasitic in man. Its home is the caecum but is occasionally found in the appendix.

white hair – greying and whitening takes place with age due to loss of pigment.

white leg – the limb becomes white, enlarged and painful. The condition can occur after childbirth. It is due to inflammation and blockage of the veins of the leg or to the spread of infection to the lymphatics of the limb through the lymphatics of the pelvis.

whites – another name for leucorrhoea.

white swelling – a name applied to tuberculous disease of joints.

whitlow – a popular term for acute inflammation of the deep seated tissues of the finger, affecting the root of the nail, the pulp of the finger tip and the sheath of the tendons that run along the back and front of the fingers.

whooping cough – a serious but preventable disease of childhood. It is especially dangerous and sometimes fatal in young infants who can readily catch the disease. It is caused by the bacteria Haemophilus pertussis and can be prevented by vaccination.

Wilm's tumour – the commonest malignant kidney tumour in the infancy occurring in 1:10,000 children. The survival rate following removal and radiotherapy is now about 80%. The tumour is otherwise called a nephroblastoma.

Wilson's disease – a familial disease caused by the increased accumulation of copper in the brain, eyes, kidneys and liver causing damage and producing symptoms as the disease progresses, such as tremor, clumsiness, psychological disturbances, weakness, emaciation, blue half-moon appearance of the nails and retraction of the upper teeth. It is also known as hepatolenticular degeneration.

winter cough – the name applied to chronic bronchitis especially affecting older people. The condition passes off and returns again the following winter.

winter vomiting disease – a condition characterised by nausea, vomiting, diarrhoea and dizziness occurring in winter (epidemic nausea and vomiting). Outbursts involve whole families and communities like schools. It is caused by a parvovirus and seldom lasts for more than 72 hours.

woolsorters disease – another name for anthrax.

word blindness – a condition in which, as a result of some disorder of the brain, a person becomes unable to associate the proper meaning with words although he may be able to spell correctly; another name sometimes but, strictly incorrectly, given to dyslexia.

word deafness – while the hearing remains perfect there is a loss of power of referring the names heard to articles they denote.

wounds – a breach suddenly in tissues of the body by direct violence.

wrist drop – dropping of the hand at the wrist with the inability to lift or extend it caused by paralysis or injury to the muscles or tendons which extend the fingers and hand (see drop wrist).

writer's cramp – spasm affecting certain muscles when engaged in writing. May not occur when the muscles are used in other activities.

wry neck – a condition in which the head is twisted to one side. It may be caused by the contraction of a scar, but in the majority of cases it is a spasmodic condition due to an excessive tendency for certain muscles to contract.

xanthelasmata – yellow plaques of fat deposited on the skin. They tend to occur on the eyelids in hyperlipidaemia.

xanthomata – deposits of fatty tissue in the tendon sheaths or over bony prominences.

xeroderma – rough dry condition of the skin with copious formation of scales.

xerosis – abnormal dryness especially of the eye.

xerostoma – dryness of the mouth due to lack of saliva.

yaws – a tropical disease caused by spirochaetes resembling the syphilis organism. It is non-venereal and may be transmitted by insect bites. It presents as fever, rheumatic pains, skin eruptions and can lead to the destruction of the skin and bones of the nose if not treated.

yellow fever – a virus infection characterised by fever and jaundice. The infection is transmitted to man by the mosquito Aedes aegypti and is endemic in tropical regions of Central and South America, West Africa. Visitors to yellow fever areas can be protected by vaccination.

> Yellow fever is usually associated with West Africa ('the white man's grave') and tropical areas of the Caribbean, Central and South America.
>
> However, at one time it was rife in some of the major cities of the U.S.A.
>
> The last city in the U.S.A. to suffer an epidemic was New Orleans in 1906. By that time the mosquito vector was known and effective control measures became available.
>
> The first detailed account of yellow fever came from Cotton Mather who, in 1693, described a disease brought to Boston on a British man-of-war as 'a most pestilential fever which carried off his neighbour with very direful symptoms of turning yellow, vomiting and bleeding in every way'.
>
> In 1807 Napoleon Bonaparte sent an army to suppress an uprising in Haiti. The uprising failed but the army was almost totally destroyed by yellow fever.

zoonosis – animal diseases which can be transmitted to man.

zoster or zona – two names for the eruption known as shingles.

> SHINGLES –
> An infection caused by the same virus as chicken pox, mainly occurring in adults. It is characterised by skin eruptions along the cutaneous nerves usually on one side of the body (particularly the girdle, thorax, face or head) and frequently accompanied by severe neuralgia. The virus may remain latent between attacks.

> The consultant stopped by the bed of a middle-aged female patient and addressing the students announced: "This is a 58-year-old lady suffering from recurrent attacks of chronic inflammation around the fallopian tubes and ovaries.
> "As a young woman she was a prostitute and had several attacks of venereal disease which needed prolonged courses of treatment at the local clinic. How far do you think her previous dissolute life is responsible for her condition today?"
> For the next 15 minutes a discussion took place over the patient, who was completely ignored.
> As the retinue moved on the lady grabbed the young house surgeon by the arm: "Insensitive bugger that consultant," she said, "Fancy mentioning my age in front of all them students."

THE HISTORY OF MEDICINE

Every day we become more conscious of our human past.

Almost every day a new discovery is made, enabling us to develop the time-sense which is essential for human development.

> 'Time present and time past
> Are both perhaps present in time future,
> And time future contained in time past.'

> (From *'Four Quartets'* by T.S. Eliot – 1888-1965)

The medical discoveries recorded from over 3,000 years before the birth of Christ to the present day are fascinating.

Does it mean that man can make himself immortal?

Can our good genes – once we have eliminated the bad ones – be preserved, transported to a distant planet of our own choice, and then re-vitalised in a new world?

And if it does become possible will we be able to take with us the works of those who were great on this tiny planet, from Aristotle onwards?

Will they be on microfiche, CD, internet? Or will they be in some sort of memory disc implanted in our heads by eminent neuro-surgeons?

Are we merely peering out of the animal world which has been our progenitor?

Was it a great big bang, or is there some Supreme Being smiling at our attempts to reach Him/Her?

In his 'Back to Methuselah' (sub-titled 'A Metabiological Pentateuch'), George Bernard Shaw started with the Garden of Eden and ended in 21,920. Anno Domini, of course.

If, and when, we do arrive, will our earthly favourites be there so that we can continue applauding, laughing, marvelling, weeping?

In the following pages we record the history of medicine, and its development to the genetic marker.

Great scientists, physicians and surgeons have made it possible for the ailments that afflict us to be alleviated. It has taken thousands of years to discover the gene markers.

As the universe has existed for many millions of years those thousands of years are dots on the development of humankind.

A CHRONOLOGICAL RECORD

BC

c2500 There is tooth filling in Sumer, in Southern Iraq. The Sumerian civilisation was established there about 5000 BC.

c1950 Physicians in Babylon and Syria base their medical practices on astrology and a belief in demons.

c1500 Contraceptives are being used in Egypt.

The Edwin Smith Surgical Papyrus is written, although it appears to be a copy of a manuscript written about 2500 BC. It is a scientific treatise on surgery.

The Papyrus Ebers gives a description of 700 medications. It also shows that physicians prescribe diets, fasting and massage, and that some practise hypnosis.

THE SCIENTIST WHO BECAME A GOD

No, not one of our modern scientists. It is an ancient one – Imhotep!

He flourished in Egypt about 3,000 years before the birth of Christ, and although he is regarded as the first scientist he was also famous as a physician.

Scientists, of course, are students or experts in one or more of the natural or physical sciences.

Their investigations are exhaustive, their findings inexhaustible, and they leave us all exhausted with their contradictions of discoveries found before them. Nevertheless, progress is essential and Imhotep, although his discoveries were the result of trial-and-error experimentation, was assigned a godly ancestry and magical properties after his death.

The fame of the Egyptian healers was so great that from all over the Middle East, and later the Mediterranean, rich and noble persons went to Egypt to be healed. Egyptian priests removed the internal organs of cadavers in order to understand the human body. To treat the still-living, mouldy bread would be put on wounds. Castor oil and poppy juices were used.

It is even recorded that the thousands who built the pyramids and temples were encouraged to eat radishes, garlic and onions because it was believed that they prevented epidemic diseases.

Many scientists now confirm that these vegetables contain ingredients which have antibiotic properties. The feminine sex may find them not so efficacious! Less likely to be efficacious was Nile mud, dung and even urine.

The Egyptians believed that gods watched over each body part, and therefore certain priests devoted themselves to a particular god and to a particular part of the body.

Surgery was different. The Edwin Smith Surgical Papyrus and the Ebers Papyrus are copies of manuscripts prepared a thousand or more years earlier.

Continued on page 126

They tell us how to set bones (learned from those taken from the cadavers?), about the pumping functions of heart, and that the pulse can be used to determine how the heart is functioning. Medications and diets are also prescribed.

Egypt became a Roman province in 30 BC, but Egyptian medicine continued to dominate the known world for some time to come.

Imhotep reigned supreme for over 3,000 years.

c1000   There is leprosy in India and Egypt.

c800   Homer refers to highly developed battlefield surgery.

c500   Alcmaeon of Croton (Greek anatomist and physician) discovers difference between veins and arteries, also connection between brain and sensing organs. He discovers Eustachian tubes and dissects human cadavers for scientific purposes. He notes the optic nerve, recognising the brain as the seat of intellect.

Susrata performs the first cataract operations in India.

c440   Greek philosopher Empedocles of Akragas (Sicily) recognises that the heart is the centre of the system of blood vessels.

c400   Hippocrates founds the profession of physicians, develops the Hippocratic oath, and encourages the separation of medicine from religion at his school of medicine at Cos. He recognised that disease had natural causes, and has earned the soubriquet 'The Father of Medicine'.

c330   Praxagoras, a Greek physician born at Cos, distinguishes between veins and arteries, although he thinks that arteries are hollow tubes that carry air throughout the body.

c290   Diocles (a student of Aristotle's) writes the first book on anatomy and the first book of herbal remedies.

Epicurus argues that organs develop through exercise and weaken when not in use.

Herophilus and Erasistratus flourish in Alexandria. They perform dissections in public, and describe the liver, spleen, retina, duodenum, ovaries, Fallopian tubes and prostate gland. They agree that the seat of learning is the brain and not the heart.

c160   Erasistratus comes very close to recognising the circulation of the blood, especially by noting the relationship of the lungs to the circulatory system.

c120   Asclepiades of Bythinia (Turkey) believes that disease, which he treats with baths, diet and exercise, is caused by a disturbance in the particles that make up the body.

c40   The Ayurveda is compiled. It becomes the basic Hindu medical treatise.

c1   Celsus, Roman medical encyclopaedist, writes of many things, but only the medical books survive. They include descriptions of surgical procedures and dentistry, and of such disorders as cataract of the eye.

THE GREAT GREEK PHILOSOPHER

Specialisation is the name of the game today.

The known universe is expanding so quickly that a new science is discovered almost every week!

Perhaps very soon we will have new sciences in every planet in the universe. However, unlike movement and communication around the earth it will be very difficult for Martian scientists to take a working holiday on the Moon or on Jupiter or Mars.

Aristotle was born in 384 BC and died in 322 BC. His world was smaller, and he was able to devote himself to logic, metaphysics, physics, astronomy, meteorology, biology, psychology, ethics, politics – and even literary criticism.

His contribution to medical thought is through his biological reasoning. He classified animals and plants. He divided animals into those with and without blood systems, and divided those with blood streams into fish, amphibians, reptiles, birds and mammals (that's us!).

Recent discoveries of live coral would give him food for thought, were he still alive.

Aristotle's work in embryology is of great importance.

He discovered that the mother is as important in procreation as the father. Before Aristotle, the common Greek notion was that the man supplied the seed and that the woman's role was rather like the soil when a seed is planted.

Will there come a time when a woman can plant her egg in a man's body and after nine months he gives birth?

> Hamlet said to Horatio:
> *"There are more things in heaven and earth, Horatio,*
> *Than are dreamt of in your philosophy".*
> Was Shakespeare thinking of Aristotle?

As he sat in the fading light with his quill pen in his hand, was he thinking of Aristotle, the Amazons and the biological change in the human mammal?

Perhaps there are more things in heaven and earth yet to come!

AD

c19 Thaddeus of Florence describes the uses of alcohol in De Virtutibus Aquae Vitae (On the Virtues of Alcohol).

c49 De Materia Medica by Greek physician Pedianius Dioscorides of Anazarbus (Turkey) deals with the medical properties of about 600 plants and nearly a thousand drugs.

c200 Galen of Pergamum (Turkey) extracts plant juices for medicinal purposes and consolidates the work of the Alexandrian doctors.

THE EMPEROR'S PHYSICIAN

Remember the gladiators? Galen (Claudius Galenus) was their chief physician in Pergamum from 157 AD. He was only 27 years of age. Then he moved to Rome and became physician to three emperors – Marcus Aurelius, Commodus and Severus.

He was the first physician to diagnose by the pulse.

Imagine those gladiators looking at him with glazed eyes, saying to him appealingly, "Am I still alive, doctor?"

And imagine Galen's encouraging reply, "Well, your heart is still beating. I'll recommend 7 days' sick leave and then you can come back and have another go!"

Galen wrote on many medical and philosophical matters, and his extant work consists of 83 genuine treatises and 15 commentaries on Hippocrates.

c541	A pandemic of the bubonic plague strikes Europe and the Empire of Justinian, killing at its peak 10,000 persons a day in Constantinople. It continues until 544.
c542	The plague in Constantinople, imported by rats from Egypt and Syria, soon spreads all over Europe.
c547	The plague reaches Britain.
c590	The plague is now in Rome.
c594	The plague ends, but not before it halves the population of Europe
c600	From India, smallpox spreads via China and Asia Minor to Southern Europe.
c643	The Chinese physician Chen Ch'uan dies. He was the first person to have noted the symptoms of diabetes mellitus, including thirst and sweet urine.
c664	There is a plague outbreak in Saxon England.
c750	There are St. Vitus' dance epidemics in Germany.
c857	The first reports of ergotism epidemics in western Europe.
c900	Phases (the Arab physician) mentions as infectious diseases: plague, consumption, smallpox, rabies. He describes them.
c977	In Baghdad a hospital is founded which employs 24 physicians and contains a surgery and a department for eye disorders.
c1021	St. Vitus epidemics in Europe.
c1123	St. Bartholomew's Hospital in London is founded.
c1140	Roger II, a Norman king, decrees that only physicians with a licence from the government may practise medicine.
c1200	Alcohol is now being used for medical purposes.
c1230	Leprosy is imported to Europe by the Crusaders.
c1303	Spectacles are being used.

c1316   Mondino de'Luzzi's Anatomia (Anatomy) is the first work devoted to human anatomy and the art of dissection to be written in the West. It is based upon the dissection of corpses.

c1329   Henri de Mondeville's Chirurgia (Surgery) advocates sutures and cleansing of wounds.

c1332   Bubonic plague originates in India.

c1347   The Black Death devastates Europe.

        By 1349 the Black Death has killed a third of the population of England.

c1351   Between 1347 and 1351 it is estimated that approximately 75 million people die of the Black Death.

c1361   The Black Death reappears in England.

c1369   Guy de Chauliac's Chirurgia Magna describes how to treat fractures and hernias.

c1377   The first quarantine station is set up in Ragusa (Dubrovnik). Those suspected of plague have to stay there for 40 days.

c1493   Christopher Columbus finds that Native Americans use tobacco as a medicine.

c1414   Influenza is recorded for the first time in Paris.

c1452   The first professional association for midwives is founded in 1452 in Regensburg (Germany).

        Nicholas of Cusa constructs spectacles for the near-sighted.

c1460   Heinrich von Pfolspeundt writes Bundt-Ertzney – the first book on surgery ever published in Germany.

c1490   In Padua (Italy) an anatomical theatre is opened for the demonstration of the dissection of corpses.

        Leonardo da Vinci notes that liquids in tubes with a small diameter tend to crawl up the tubes, taking the first notice of capillary action.

c1495   A syphilis epidemic spreads from beleaguered Naples all over Europe through French soldiers.

        The French army of Charles VIII takes Naples. Camp defenders of the defending Spaniards infect his troops with syphilis, possibly brought from the Americas by Columbus' sailors. Then some of the army move back to France, infecting the Italian peninsular and northern Europe.

c1497   Hieronymus Brunschwygk publishes the first known book on the surgical treatment of gunshot wounds.

c1499   Benedetto Rinio's Liber de Implicius, describes and illustrates 400 plants that have medicinal uses.

c1500   Hieronymous Brunschwygk's Liber de Arte Distillandi de Simplicibus, known as 'The Small Book', describes the construction of furnaces and stills, herbs usable for distillation, and medical applications of distillates. Then he publishes his 'Big Book' dealing with the same subjects.

        Jakop Nufer of Switzerland performs the first recorded Caesarean operation on a living woman.

c1518   Spectacles are being used for the shortsighted.

        Smallpox reaches the Americas, causing a major epidemic among the Indians of the island of Hispaniola.

c1518 The Royal College of Physicians in London is established.

c1519 Andreas Caesalpinus is born in Italy. He anticipated William Harvey's theory of blood circulation.

c1520 A smallpox epidemic among the Aztec demoralises them and helps Fernando Cortes and a small band of Spaniards (immune to the disease from child exposure) to take over the Aztec empire.

Phillipus Aureolus Paracelsus (Theophrastrus Bombast von Hohenheim) introduces tincture of opium, which he names laudanum.

c1525 Smallpox kills Huayna Capac, the ruler of the Incas.

c1528 Severe outbreaks of the plague in England.

c1529 In Padua, Giovanni Battista da Monte (Italian physician) introduces clinical examinations of patients at the sickbed.

c1530 Girolamo Fracastoro's 'Syphilis Sive de Morbo Gallico' (On Syphilis, or the French Disease) describes the symptoms, spread and treatment. He coins the word syphilis, which is the name of a young shepherd who develops the disease.

Paracelsus's Paragranum argues that medicine should be based upon nature and its physical laws. He is the first to suggest the use of chemical substances, such as compounds of mercury and antimony, as remedies.

c1533 The first lunatic asylums are opened (without medical attention).

c1542 A book on anatomy by Jean Francois Fernel (France) is the first to describe appendicitis and peristalsis (the waves of contraction in the digestive system that move food through the alimentary canal).

THE
ALL ROUND GENIUS

All rounders are rare. All round geniuses are even more rare.

Aristotle was one.

Leonardo da Vinci was another.

They were divided by over a millenium – 1,200 years!

A genius can be brilliant in a particular sphere: Cezanne in art, Beethoven and Mozart in musical expression, Shakespeare in dramatic poetry, Rodin and Henry Moore in sculpture.

Geniuses who can reveal a broader conceptual range are rare.

Da Vinci was a real genius. He was a great artist, and at the same time had a wide understanding of the sciences which included biology, anatomy, physiology, hydro-dynamics, mechanics and even aeronautics!

His writings contain original remarks on all these subjects.

c1543 Flemish anatomist Andreas Vesalius writes the first accurate work on the human anatomy: De Humani Corporis Fabrica (On the Structure of the Human Body).

c1544 St Bartholomew's Hospital in London is refounded.

c1545 A book on surgery by Ambroise Paré (France) advocates abandoning the practice of treating wounds with boiling oil and using soothing ointments instead.

c1546 Girolamo Fracastoro (in his De Contagione – On Contagion) advances the idea that diseases are seedlike entities that are transferred from person to person.

c1552 Italian anatomist Bartolomeo Eustachio describes the adrenal glands, the detailed structure of the teeth, and the Eustachian tubes (named after him). His work is not published until 1714.

King Edward VI founds Christ's Hospital in London.

c1553 Michael Servetus's anonymously published book on theology contains his view that blood circulates from the heart to the lungs and back. He is discovered, and he is burned at the stake in Geneva by John Valcin.

c1559 Italian anatomist Realdo Colombo supports Galen against the new anatomy of Vesalius. However, he demonstrates that Galen was wrong about the way blood travels from the heart to the lungs and back. In his De Re Anatomica (Of Anatomical Matters) he claims that blood circulates from the right chamber of the heart to the lungs and then to the left chamber. Galen thought the blood passed directly between the two chambers.

c1561 Italian anatomist Gabriel Fallopius, in his Observationes Anatomicae (Anatomical Observations) describes the organs of the inner ear and the female reproductive system, including the Fallopian tubes named after him.

c1562 There is a plague in Paris.

Pierre Franco (famous French surgeon) dies. He has performed bladder and cataract operations.

c1563 General outbreak of plague in Europe kills over 20,000 people in London.

c1567 Two million Indians die in South America of typhoid fever.

c1575 There are outbreaks of plague in Sicily, spreading through Italy up to Milan.

c1579 Glass eyes are now being made!

c1592 A plague kills 15,000 people in London.

c1601 Many 'Badestuben' (German brothels) are closed by the authorities because of the spread of venereal disease.

c1603 There is a heavy outbreak of plague in England.

Hieronymus Fabricius's De Venarium Ostiolis (On the Valves in the Veins) presents a detailed study of valves in veins.

c1604 One of the first important studies in embryology, De Formata Foetu (On the Format of the Foetus) by Hieronymus Fabricius ab Aguappendente (Italy) contains a study of blood circulation in the umbilical cord.

c1614 The first study of metabolism is in Sanctorius Sanctorius's De Statica Medicina. He measures changes in his own weight, pulse and temperature.

c1616   William Harvey lectures about the circulation of the blood to the Royal College of Physicians in England.

c1619   William Harvey announces at St. Bartholomew's Hospital, London, his discovery of the circulation of the blood.

c1624   Thomas Sydenham is born in Wynford Eagle in England. He is called 'The English Hippocrates' and is the first to describe measles and to identify scarlet fever. He advocates the use of opium to relieve pain, chinchona bark (quinine) to relieve malaria, and iron to relieve anaemia.

c1626   Sanctorius Sanctorius (Italian physician) measures human temperature with a thermometer for the first time.

c1628   William Harvey publishes Exerticatio Anatomica de Motu Cordis et Sanguinis in Animalibus (Anatomical Treatise on the Movement of the Heart and Blood in Animals) which describes his discovery of the circulation of the blood.

c1631   Richard Lower, born near Bodmin, England, observes that contact with air turns dark blood from the veins bright. He establishes the fact that phlegm does not, as Galen had claimed, originate in the brain.

c1639   Quinine is being used for medicinal purposes.

c1641   Arsenic is being prescribed for medicinal purposes.

c1647   There is yellow fever in Barbados.

Jean Pecquet (France) discovers the thoracic duct.

c1655   Johann Shultes's Armementarium Chirugicum (The Hardware of the Surgeon) describes a procedure for removing a human breast.

1657   William Harvey dies on June 3rd.

c1658   Jan Swammerdam (Holland) is the first to see and describe red blood cells.

Sir Thomas Browne (1605-1682), an English physician, advocates cremation.

c1659   Thomas Willis (English physician) describes first typhoid fever

c1660   Marcello Malpighi (Italy) shows that lungs consist of many small air pockets and a complex system of blood vessels. By observing capillaries through a microscope he completes the work of Harvey in describing the circulation of the blood.

Edme Mariotte (France) discovers the blind spot in the eye.

c1664   Thomas Willis's Cerebri Anatome (Anatomy of the Brain) is the most complete and accurate account of the brain and nervous system put forward to date.

c1665   In De Cerebro, Malpighi describes how the nervous system consists of bundles of fibres connected to the brain by the spinal cord.

Peter Chamberlain, court physician to Charles II, invents midwifery forceps.

The Great Plague of London

c1667   Robert Boyle demonstrates before the Royal Society that an animal can be kept alive by artificial respiration.

Thomas Willis's Pathologiae Cerebri (Pathology of the Brain) is the first account of the effects of the late stage of syphilis on the brain (although Willis does not recognise the cause of these symptoms).

AN OPEN LETTER

To: Dr. William Harvey, St. Bartholomew's Hospital, London.

Dear Doctor,

You will not have heard of me, because this is written about 350 years after you died in 1657.

The reason why I am writing is because it appears that you discovered how the blood circulated through the human body, and published your findings in Exercitatio Anatomica de Motu Cordis et Sanguinis which you published in 1628.

You set up your practice as a physician in 1602, and you were appointed physician to St. Bartholomew's Hospital in 1609.

You were only 31 years of age.

Now, hundreds of years later, with private aeroplanes, the Concorde, helicopters, motorways and all those Mercs about, it is difficult to appreciate how you managed to get from one place to another with important medical matters on your mind.

For example, doctor, you were physician to James I and Charles I.

What secrets did James tell you about his mother, Mary Queen of Scots? And how did you get on with his views about the divine right of kings?

In 1636 you accompanied the Earl of Arundel to Nuremberg and demonstrated your theory on blood circulation there.

And what about Charles I? You attended him at the battle of Edgehill in 1642, and then accompanied him to Oxford as warden of Merton College.

If you are still around, up there in the firmament, I hope you can read this open letter. Your works were published in Latin in 1766, so you may not easily appreciate this modern approach.

The circulation of the blood is of paramount importance to us.

Since you 'retired' in 1657 a great deal of work has been undertaken by physicians and surgeons, and I'm sure they are as grateful as we all are because you were able to explain how the blood circulation works.

Your book on animal reproduction Exercitaciones de Generatione Animalium, published in 1651, indicates how passionately involved you were in the blood circulatory system of the animal world. Presumably you then felt that we humans were also animals.

I wonder where you were on 7th February, when Charles I lost his head as he had never lost it before?

In 1767 Voltaire wrote in his L'Ingenu: "Indeed, history is nothing more than a tableau of crimes and misfortunes."

Executing Charles I was a crime. Not making you a Lord (or at least a Knight of the Realm) was a misfortune. Nowadays you might have become a Lord! Lesser mortals have!

F.C.

c1669   There is an outbreak of cholera in China.

Richard Lower's Tractacus de corde describes the structure of the heart and its properties as a muscle, and notes that blood changes colour in the lungs.

c1670   Thomas Willis announces his rediscovery of the connection between sugar in the urine and diabetes mellitus (a connection already known to the Greeks, the Chinese and the Indians).

c1673   Malpighi's De Formatione Pulli (on the formation of the chick in the egg) describes the development of the ovum.

c1675   Nicolaus Steno demonstrates that eggs are formed inside the dogfish before it gives birth to live offspring. He leaps to the conclusion that mammals have eggs. Regnier de Graaf had reached the same conclusion earlier.

c1676   There is an influenza epidemic in England.

c1677   Anton van Leeuwenhoek discovers protozoa. He concludes that sperm are the source of reproduction. He also discovers the microscope.

c1681   The Chelsea Hospital in London is founded for wounded and discharged soldiers.

c1683   Anton van Leeuwenhoek observes bacteria. It will not be seen by other scientists for more than a century.

c1691   Clopton Havers (England) publishes the first complete textbook on the bones of the human body.

John Ray's 'The Wisdom of God Manifested in the Works of Creation' suggests that fossils are the remains of animals from the distant past. Ray is established as the leader of the natural history movement in England.

c1693   John Ray's 'Synopsis Animalium Quadrupedem et Serpentini' (A General View of Four-legged Animals and Snakes) introduces the first important classification of animals. It follows Aristotle's divisions into 'blooded' and 'bloodless', and correctly classifies whales as mammals.

c1700   Bernadino Rammazzini's 'De Morbis Artificum' is the first systematic treatment of occupational disorders. He concludes that more nuns than married women develop breast cancer, possibly for reasons related to pregnancy and lactation.

c1701   Giacomo Pylarini, considered by some to be the first immunologist, inoculates three children with smallpox in Constantinople. He hopes to prevent their developing more serious cases of smallpox when they are older.

c1704   Antonio Maria Valsalva (Italy) in his 'De Aure Humana Tractatus' (Anatomy and Disease of the Ear) provides the first detailed description of the physiology of the ear.

c1705   Raymond Vieussens (France) gives the first accurate description of the left ventricle of the heart, the valve of the large coronary vein, and the course of coronary blood vessels.

c1707   John Floyer (England) introduces the physician's pulse watch, which counts the pulse rate.

c1707 Giovanni Maria Lanccisi (Italy) offers the first discussion of cardiac pathology in his 'De Subitaneis Mortibus' (On Sudden Death).

c1708 Hermann Boerhaave (Holland) explains his theory of inflammation. 'Institutiones Medicae' combines mechanical views of physiology with the idea that physiological processes are chemical fermentations.

c1710 The Berlin Charité (Hospital) is founded.

c1711 Luigi Marsigli shows the animal nature of corals, formerly believed to be plants.

c1717 Lady Mary Wortley Montagu introduces inoculation against smallpox in England.

Giovannie Lancisi suggests in 'De Noxiis Palludum Effluviss' (On the Noxious Effluvia of Marshes) that malaria can be transmitted by a mosquito.

THE FAMOUS HUNTER BROTHERS

William Hunter (1817-1783), the Scottish anatomist and obstetrician was born in Long Calderwood, East Kilbride, and his brother John (a physiologist and surgeon) was born 10 years later.

Their father was a younger son of the ancient house of Hunterston, in Ayrshire. William studied divinity for five years, but was then trained in anatomy at St. George's Hospital in London. He confined himself to midwifery, and in 1764 he was appointed physician-extraordinary to Queen Charlotte Sophia.

He was the first Professor of Anatomy at the Royal Academy. He built a house with an amphitheatre for lectures, a dissecting room and a museum, and bequeathed the museum to Glasgow University.

His brother John studied surgery at Chelsea Hospital and St. Bartholomew's and then became house-surgeon at St. George's Hospital.

One of his students was Edward Jenner, and in 1776 he was appointed surgeon-extraordinary to King George III.

In 1790 be became surgeon-general to the army, and after a long and distinguished career he died in 1793, and is buried in Westminster Abbey.

---

c1719 Westminster Hospital is founded in London.

c1721 Zabstiel Boylston introduces inoculation against smallpox into America during the Boston epidemic.

Jean Palfyn introduces the use of forceps for facilitating birth.

c1722 Thomas Guy (a London bookseller) dedicates £300,000 for founding Guy's Hospital.

c1730 Reaumur constructs an alcohol thermometer with a graduated scale.

George Martini performs the first tracheotomy for treatment of diphtheria.

c1736 Claudius Aymand performs the first successful operation for appendicitis.

William Douglass (American physician) describes scarlet fever.

c1739 The Foundling Hospital is established in London.

c1740 There is a smallpox epidemic in Berlin.

c1745 The Middlesex Hospital is founded in England.

c1747 Bernhard Siegfried Allbinus' 'Tabula Sceleti et Musculorem Corporis Humani' (Plates of the Skeleton and Muscles of the Human Body) shows relative parts of bones and muscles in correct proportions.

The first textbook on physiology is produced by Albrecht von Haller (Switzerland). It's called 'Primae Lineae Physiologgiae'.

c1748 John Fothergill (England) gives the first description of diphtheria in his 'Account of the Putrid Throat'.

HE VACCINATED AN 8-YEAR-OLD BOY!

It was Edward Jenner (1749-1823), an English physician.

He studied under John Hunter in London, then settled in Berkeley, Gloucestershire, close to the home where he was born.

In 1775 he began to examine the truth of the traditions respecting cowpox, becoming convinced that it was efficacious as a protection against smallpox.

The crowning experiment was made in 1796, when he vaccinated an 8-year-old boy with cowpox matter from the hands of a milkmaid, and shortly afterwards inoculated him with smallpox.

There was violent opposition for a year, until surgeons and physicians in London signed a declaration of their entire confidence in it.

c1752 William Smellie's Treatise on midwifery is the first scientific approach to obstetrics.

Manchester Royal Infirmary is founded.

c1754 The University of Halle (Germany) graduates the first female with a degree of medical doctor.

c1760 The first British school for the deaf and dumb is opened by Thomas Braidwood at Edinburgh, Scotland.

c1761 Giovanni Morgagni's 'De Sedibus et Causis Morborum per Anatomen Indagatis' (On the Causes of Diseases) is the first important work in pathological anatomy.

c1763 The first American medical society is founded in New London.

c1764 Robert Whytt's 'Observations on Nervous, Hypochondriacal, or Hysteric Diseases' is the first important textbook on neurology

c1765 Robert Whytt's 'Observations on the Dropsy of the Brain' gives the first description of tuberculosis meningitis in children.

c1768 John Hunter begins the foundation of experimental and surgical pathology.

c1771 New York Hospital is founded.

c1772 Italian anatomist Antonia Scarpa discovers the labyrinth of the ear – the semi-circular canals, vestibule and cochlea.

c1774   William Hunter (Scotland) produces 'Anatomy of the Human Gravid Uterus', containing masterpieces of anatomical illustration.

Mesmer (Austrian physician) uses hypnosis for health purposes.

ARE YOU ANIMALICALLY MAGNETIC?

Do you have some special chemical attraction?

If you have, whom do you attract?

Do dogs lick your hand? Do cats look at you mournfully, and then slink off into the night?

Does your eyeball contact hold or is eyeball contact difficult?

Are you easily hypnotised?

The founder of mesmerism was Friedrich Anton Mesmer (1734-1815). He was an Austrian physician and a founder of mesmerism. He was born near Constance, and studied and practised medicine at Vienna.

It was around 1772, when he was 38, that Mesmer took up the idea that there existed a power which he called 'animal magnetism'.

In 1778 he went to Paris and created a sensation by curing diseases at seances. No doubt his 'patients' wanted to be cured. He was denounced as an impostor and retired to obscurity.

Can you mesmerise? Can you command the attention of your Rottweiler, your poodle, or your Siamese cat? That would be pure animal magnetism.

Mesmer must have made quite an impact during his time or the word mesmerism would not be in our dictionaries.

Mesmerism led to hypnotism, and it was used by entertainers and charlatans until the UK Hypnosis Act of 1952 controlled its exploitation. Hypnosis is used to treat disorders such as addictions to tobacco or overeating.

It has been tried on footballers, but presumably if you have a split second in which to decide whether you should shoot or pass the ball to a colleague, your hypnotist would not have time to advise you.

Try auto-suggestion and shoot, man! Shoot!

c1775   Sir Percival Potts suggests that chimney sweeps in London develop cancers of the scrotum and of the nasal cavity as a result of exposure to soot. It is the first suggestion that environmental factors can cause cancer.

William Withering (England) introduces digitalis to cure the dropsy associated with heart disease.

c1778   John Hunter's 'A Practical Treatise on the Diseases of the Teeth' classifies teeth into molars, bicuspids, cuspids and incisors.

Mesmer practises 'mesmerism' in Paris.

c1779   In London the first children's clinic is opened.

c1784   In Paris the first school for the blind is opened.

c1786   Benjamin Rush's 'Observations on the Cause and Cure of the Tetanus' suggests that some illnesses may be psychosomatic.

c1790 Marshall Hall (England), physiologist, is the first to identify and study reflexes. Later he denounces bloodletting as a treatment for disease.

c1793 Jean-Pierre-Marie Flourens (France) studies the nervous system, locates the centre of respiration, and demonstrates that the cerebellum controls muscular movements.

c1795 Matthew Baillie (Scotland) publishes 'Morbid Anatomy of Some of the Most Important Parts of the Human Body'. It is the first work to treat pathology as a subject in itself.

Sir Gilbert Blane (Scotland), a physician, uses lime juice to prevent scurvy in the British Navy. It is the origin of the nickname 'Limey' for the British sailor.

c1796 Edward Jenner (England) performs the first vaccination against smallpox by infecting a body with cowpox (vaccinia virus).

c1797 The Royal Society rejects Jenner's vaccination technique for smallpox.

c1798 Edward Jenner publishes his work on vaccination.

c1800 William Cruikshank (England) uses chlorine to purify water.

Benjamin Waterhouse (USA) uses smallpox vaccine on his own son.

Humphrey Davy (England) discovers nitrous oxide (laughing gas) and suggests it can be used as an anaesthetic.

OPEN WIDE!

Sir Humphrey Davy (1778-1829) was a wood-carver's son and became a chemist. While employed with Thomas Beddoes as an assistant at his Medical Pneumatic Institution he experimented with various newly-discovered gases.

It was then that he discovered the anaesthetic effect of laughing-gas, nitrous oxide. Although he suggested its possible use in surgical anaesthesia, this was not followed up until 1844 when Horace Wells, a dentist from Hartford, Connecticut, used the gas for extracting teeth in his practice. Unfortunately the use of nitrous oxide fell into disrepute when Wells' demonstration of its use, at Harvard Medical School, was a failure. By the time it was used again in anaesthesia, ether and chloroform had come into use.

Davy invented a safe lamp for use in gassy coalmines, quite apart from being ahead of his time in wishing to encourage us to laugh at the dentist as he extracts our incisors and molars.

---

c1801 Thomas Young (England) discovers the cause of astigmatism.

c1804 Kark Rokitansky (Austria), pathologist, through dissecting more than 30,000 cadavers, is the first to recognise many pathological changes caused through disease, and is the first to discover bacteria as the cause of malignant endocarditis.

c1805 Franz Joseph Gall shows that different parts of the brain have different functions, but makes the mistake of explaining that the brain can be studied by examining the shape of a person's skull – phrenology.

c1810 Samuel Friedrich Hahnemann's 'Organon of Rational Healing' introduces homeopathy.

Charles Bell publishes 'New Anatomy of the Brain', in which he discusses the difference between sensory and motor nerves. The anterior (spinal) roots are motor, and posterior roots are sensory.

c1811 Samuel Hahnemann publishes his catalogue of homeopathic drugs.

c1812 Benjamin Rush (England) publishes 'Medical Enquiries and Observations upon the Diseases of the Mind'. It contains one of the first modern attempts to explain mental disorders.

c1815 Carl Reinhold Wunderlich (Germany) is the first to realise that taking accurate temperatures of patients with a thermometer is useful.

c1816 Theophile Rene Laennec (France) invents the stethoscope.

c1817 James Parkinson (England) writes an essay on 'The Shaking Palsy'. It gives a clinical description of the disease which now bears his name.

c1818 Jean-Baptiste Dumas (France) treats goitre with iodine.

c1819 Theophile Rene Laennec publishes 'Traite de l'Auscultation Mediate' (Treatise on Diagnosis by Listening to Sounds). The stethoscope can be used to investigate lungs, heart and liver.

c1821 Charles Bell gives the first description of facial paralysis, known as Bell's palsy.

c1822 William Beaumont (Lebanon) starts an experimental study of digestion in the exposed stomach of a wounded man.

c1823 The British Medical Journal 'The Lancet' is now published.

c1824 Charles Bell's Injuries of the Spine and Thigh Bone is published.

Henry Hickman uses carbon dioxide on an animal as a general anaesthetic.

c1825 Pierre Bretonnau (France) successfully performs the first tracheotomy to restore breathing to a child suffering from diphtheria.

Max Johann Sigismund Schultze (German anatomist) studies cytoplasm, then known as protoplasm, and shows that it is approximately the same for all forms of life.

c1826 Pierre Bretonneau describes the symptoms of diphtheria.

Karl Gegenbaur (German anatomist) shows that all vertebrate cells arise from divisions of the egg and the sperm.

c1827 Richard Bright (England) describes the symptoms of Bright's disease, a kidney disorder.

c1829 The first text on pathology anatomy is written by William E. Horner and is published in the United States.

In his 'Analysis of the Phenomena of the Human Mind' James Mill tries to show that the mind is nothing more than a machine without any creative function.

Johann Schonlein describes haemophilia, a blood disorder.

c1830 Charles Bell's 'Nervous System of the Human Body' distinguishes different types of nerves.

c1831 A cholera epidemic starts in Europe and lasts for over a year.

Chloroform is discovered by Samuel Guthrie (American chemist and physician).

The great cholera pandemic, which began in India 1826, spreads from Russia into central Europe, reaching Scotland in 1832.

c1832 The Warburton Anatomy Act legalises the sale of bodies for dissection in England. It ends the practice of body snatching and sometimes murder to provide bodies.

Thomas Hodgkin gives a description of Hodgkin's disease, a cancer of the lymph nodes.

c1833 In his 'Handbuch der Physiologie' Johannes Peter Muller (German physiologist) summarises physiological research of the period. It contains the theory that each nerve has its own specific energy.

c1834 Amalgam (mercury alloy) is used to fill teeth.

c1836 Heinrich Wilhelm Gottfried von Waldeyer-Hartz (German anatomist) is the first to note that the nervous system is built from separate cells, and that the nerve cells do not actually touch each other. He also coins the word 'chromosome'.

c1839 Charles Darwin's 'Journal of Researches into the Geology and Natural History of the Various Countries Visited by HMS Beagle, 1832-1836' is an account of Darwin's work as a scientist, principally in South America, where he collects fossils, plants and animals, and studies the geology of the continent.

c1840 Friedrich Gustav Jakob Henle (German pathologist and anatomist) expresses in his 'Pathologischen Untersuchungen' his conviction that diseases are transmitted by living organisms, but no hard evidence is offered.

c1841 Charles Thomas Jackson (America) discovers that ether is an anaesthetic.

Emile Theodor Kocher (Swiss surgeon) develops surgical removal of the thyroid as a cure for goiter.

c1842 Crawford Williamson Long (America) uses ether in surgery.

c1843 Emil Heinrich du Bois-Reymond (Germany) demonstrates that electricity is used by the nervous system to communicate between different parts of the body.

Oliver Wendell Holmes (America) advises doctors to prevent spreading puerperal (or childbed) fever by washing their hands and wearing clean clothes. It was a common disease of mothers after childbirth.

Sir David Ferrier (Scottish neurologist) uses brains of living primates and other animals to locate motor and sensory regions and to map them.

c1844 A connection between dirt and epidemic disease is established by 'The Commission for Enquiring into the State of Large Towns'.

Charles Thomas Jackson suggests using ether to deaden pain to a dentist, Willliam Thomas Green Morton.

Horace Wells is the first to use nitrous oxide as an anaesthetic in dentistry.

c1844 Sir Patrick Manson (Scottish physician and specialist in tropical medicine) studies elephantiasis, and is the first to suggest that the mosquito may be the vector in malaria.

c1845 Leukemia is described by Randolph Carl Virchow (Polish physician and pathologist).

c1846 In the Faroe Islands there is a measles epidemic. Peter Panum's study of how the disease progresses from person to person and from island to island is a classic on epidemiology.

Sir James Simpson (Scotland) discovers that chloroform is a better anaesthetic than ether or nitrous oxide. He uses chloroform in childbirth. His account of a new anaesthetic agent describes his discovery.

QUEEN VICTORIA USED HIS CHLOROFORM

The Scottish obstetrician was born in Bathgate in 1811. In 1840 he became professor of midwifery at Edinburgh.

It was James Young Simpson, who originated the use of ether as anaesthetic in childbirth in 1847.

He experimented on himself in the search for a better anaesthetic, and discovered the required properties in chloroform. Despite medical and religious opposition he championed its use, and when Queen Victoria used it for the birth of Prince Leopold in 1853 it was generally accepted.

The administration was then called 'chloroform à la reine'

Now Sir James Simpson, he founded gynaecology, championed hospital reform, and in 1847 he became physician to the Queen in Scotland.

c1846 Granville Hall (American psychologist) establishes the first experimental psychology laboratory in the USA at John Hopkins University.

c1847 The American Medical Association is founded.

Karl Friedrich Wilhelm Ludwig (Germany) develops a device that continously records blood pressure which he uses to show that the circulation of the blood is purely mechanical. No mysterious vital processes outside of ordinary physics need to be invoked.

c1848 Rudolph Cark Virchow coins the terms 'thrombosis' for the formation of blood clots, and 'embolus' for a blood clot that may detach and block blood vessels.

c1849 Pernicious anaemia is described by Thomas Addison (England).

The anthrax bacillus is discovered by Aloys-Antoine Pollender.

c1851 Claude Bernard (France) discovers that nerves controlling the dilation of the blood vessels control the body's temperature in humans.

The ophthalmoscope is invented by Hermann Ludwig von Helmholtz.

c1853 Alexander Wood uses hypodermic syringe for subcutaneous injections.

c1855 Florence Nightingale introduces hygienic standards into military hospitals during the Crimean War.

c1855 The third known pandemic of bubonic plague (the others started in 541AD and 1346AD) begins in China.

Thomas Addison describes the hormone deficiency disease that results from the adrenal gland. The disease is named after him.

c1856 Glycogen is discovered by Claude Bernard. It is used by the body to store glucose. When glucose is needed for energy the liver converts the glycogen back to glucose.

Edmund Wilson (Swiss zoologist) studies how fertilised eggs develop into embryos, and is the first to note the X and Y chromosomes of mammals.

c1857 Gregor Johann Mendel (Poland) starts the experiments with peas in his garden that will lead to his working out the laws of heredity.

DARWIN AND MENDEL

What a remarkable coincidence!

Gregor Mendel, a monk, and son of a peasant farmer, studied science at Vienna (1851-53). He had already been ordained a priest in 1847, and became an abbot in 1868.

In the monastery garden he discovered that the plants had inheritance characteristics. The edible peas attracted him in particular, and led to the formulation of his 'Mendel's Law of Segregation' and his 'Law of Independent Assortment.'

His principle of factorial inheritance and the quantitive investigation of single characters have become the basis of modern genetics. His laws described the mechanism by which many traits pass from generation to generation even though it was the simple pea which proved his point.

Meanwhile Charles Darwin (1809-1892) was thinking deeply in his garden at Downe, Kent, about inter-breeding, and the problem of the origin of the species. This was the great work of his life.

Darwin had already sailed in HMS Beagle, visiting Tenerife, The Cape Verde Islands, Brazil, Montevideo, Tierra del Fuego, Buenos Aires, Valparaiso, Chile, The Galapagos, Tahiti, New Zealand, Tasmania and the Keeling Islands.

It was not until November 1859 that he was able to condense his vast mass of notes and publish his great work on 'The Origin of Species by Means of Natural Selection'.

Biologists have accepted it. It is still to be accepted by others, disturbed by its implications. Perhaps the peas have it!

c1858 Franciscus Cornelis Donders (Netherlands) discovers that farsightedness can be caused by too shallow eyeballs.

The publication of 'Beitrage der Sinneswahrnehmungen' (Contribution to the Theory of Sensory Perception) is commenced by Wilhelm Wundt (German psychologist). It introduces concept of experimental psychology and becomes one of the founding works of psychology as a science.

c1859 Charles Darwin's 'On the Origin of Species by Means of Natural Selection or the Preservation of Favoured Races in the Struggle for Life' (known as The Origin of Species)' explains in detail his principle of natural selection and its influence on the evolution of different species.

1860 The Food and Drugs Act is enacted in Britain.

c1861 Psychology is presented as an exact science by Gustav Theodor Fechner's 'Elemente der Psychophysik'.

Broca's area demonstrates that a particular region is connected to a particular faculty through Pierre-Paul Broca discovering a lesion in the brain during an autopsy on a man who could not speak intelligibly.

Karl von Voit (German Physiologist) demonstrates that different foods do not provide energy for different body functions. Proteins break down at the same speed whether or not work is being done.

c1863 Louis Pasteur discovers the micro-organism responsible for the souring of wine.

Etienne-Jules Maray (French physiologist) invents the sphygmograph, the predecessor of the sphygmometer used to measure blood pressure today.

c1864 Franciscus Cornelis Donders discovers that astigmatism is caused by an uneven curvature of the lens or cornea of the eye.

c1865 Joseph Lister (England) introduces phenol as a disinfectant in surgery, reducing the surgical death rate from 45% to 15%.

FATHER OF ANTISEPTIC SURGERY

Joseph Lister was the son of the microscopist, Joseph Jackson Lister.

He revolutionised modern surgery by his introduction in 1867 of the antiseptic system. After graduating in arts and medicine, Lister became house surgeon at Edinburgh Royal Infirmary. He became regius professor of surgery at Glasgow, professor of clinical surgery at Edinburgh and at King's College Hospital, London.

He was made President of the Royal Society and was created Baron Lister of Lyme Regis in 1897, receiving the Order of Merit in 1902.

c1865 Jean-Antoine Villeman shows that tuberculosis is a contagious disease.

Joesph Lister initiates antiseptic surgery by using carbolic acid on a wound.

c1866 Mendel publishes his 'Law of Heredity'. No attention will be given to it until 1900.

c1866 Sir Thomas Clifford Allbutt (England) develops the clinical thermometer. Previously, thermometers had been very long and it had taken about 20 minutes to determine the temperature.

William Budd (England) demonstrates that limiting the contamination of a town's water supply can stop a cholera epidemic. John Snow (see page 25) had recognised this earlier

c1867 Wilhelm Wundt teaches the first course on physiological psychology at Heidelberg.

c1868 Sir Francis Galton shows that mental abilities of human beings form a normal distribution, lying along a familiar bell-shaped curve.

c1869 Paul Langerhans (German physician) makes a careful dissection of the pancreas. He discovers the small groups of cells – now called the islets of Langerhans. It is discovered later that these groups of cells are the source of insulin.

c1871 Darwin's 'The Descent of Man and Selection in Relation to Sex' discusses evidence of evolution of human beings from lower forms of life, comparing people to animals.

Walter Bradford Cannon (American physiologist) devises the use of bismuth compounds to make soft internal organs visible on X-rays.

c1872 Darwin's 'Expressions of the Emotions in Man and Animals' characterises emotion in evolutionary terms and argues that emotions are the result of the inheritance of behaviour from animals.

Jean Martin Charcot (French physician) uses hypnosis as part of his treatment for therapy. Later in 1885 Sigmund Freud is a student of Charcot's and learns this use of hypnotism from him!

c1873 Wilhelm Wundt begins publication of what is considered the most important book in the history of psychology: 'Grundzuge der Physiologischen Psychologie' (Principles of Physiological Psychology).

c1874 Franz Bretano dissents strongly with William Wundt, and publishes 'Psychologie vom Empirischen Standpunkt' (Psychology from an Empirical Standpoint).

Schack August Steenberg Krogh (Danish physiologist) discovers that capillaries in muscles are partially closed when a muscle is resting, and that the capillaries control blood flow in various parts of the body.

A. T. Still (America) founds osteopathy in Kansas.

c1875 The London Medical School for Women is founded.

c1876 Wilhelm (Willy) Friedrich Kuhne (German physiologist) discovers the enzyme trypsin in pancreatic juice and invents the term enzyme to distinguish those compounds that work equally well outside the cell as in it. He reserves the older name ferment for vital processes in cells.

c1877 Darwin's 'Biographical Sketch of an Infant', the diary of the development of his own son, is the first source of child psychology.

Robert Koch develops a way of obtaining pure cultures of bacteria.

THE GERMAN PIONEER

In 1882 he discovered the tubercle bacillus.

He had practised medicine at Hanover, but his work on wounds, septicaemia and splenic fever won him recognition in 1880.

In 1883 he led the German expedition sent to Egypt and India in search of the cholera germ.

This distinguished physician and pioneer bacteriologist won the Nobel prize for physiology or medicine in 1905.

He was Robert Koch

c1877 Louis Pasteur notes that some bacteria die when cultured with certain other bacteria, indicating that one bacterium gives off substances that kill the other. Not until 1939 is this observation put to use, when Rene Jules Dubos discovers the first antibiotics produced by a bacterium.

c1878 Paul Bert (French physiologist) announces that dissolved nitrogen in the blood of people working under pressurised air causes the disease commonly known as the 'bends' or caisson disease. He proposes that if air pressure is lowered by stages the disease will be prevented.

c1879 Louis Pasteur discovers by accident that weakened cholera bacteria fail to cause disease in chickens, and that chickens previously infected with the weakened virus are immune to the normal form of the virus, thus paving the way for the development of vaccines against many diseases – not just smallpox.

Wilhelm Wundt founds the first laboratory for psychology in Leipzig (Germany).

Albert Neisser (German physician) discovers the bacterium that causes gonorrhea.

c1880 Sigmund Freud (Austria) hears from Josef Breuer (Austria) of the hypnotic treatment of a patient suffering from psychological disabilities, and begins similar treatment for his own patients.

Louis Pasteur's 'On the Extension of the Germ Theory to the Aetiology of Certain Diseases' develops the germ theory of disease. He also demonstrates his findings on vaccination to the Academy of Medicine.

c1881 Ferdinand Cohn's 'Bacteria, the Smallest of Living Organisms' relates his pioneering work in bacteriology.

Carlos Finlay suggests that the mosquito is the carrier of yellow fever.

Edwin Klebs detects the typhoid bacillus.

Pasteur develops the first artificially produced vaccine against anthrax, a deadly disease that affects both animals and humans.

1881   Louis Pasteur (on May 5th) successfully demonstrates that vaccination of sheep and cattle against anthrax prevents their falling ill with the disease after injection with live bacteria. Unvaccinated animals die when given the same amount of live bacteria

LOUIS PASTEUR, THE GERM THEORIST

It was in the middle of the nineteenth century that some surgeons realised doctors could spread disease from one person to another.

Joseph Lister (in 1865) proposed using carbolic acid (phenol) on patients' wounds during surgery.

John Snow, a London doctor, noticed that cholera cases clustered where people used water from particular sources. He persuaded the authorities to remove a particular pump handle from a well at the centre of the largest outbreak area with the result that the number of cases in that area dropped immediately.

William Budd learned of Snow's success and repeated it in Bristol in 1866, thus stopping a potential cholera epidemic.

Louis Pasteur had shown that antiseptics could stop the spread of a disease of silkworms.

From silkworms Pasteur moved to the French army surgeons during the Franco-Prussian War of 1870. He urged them to sterilise their instruments. And they did!

He started with anthrax, and then discovered that vaccination with a weakened bacteria could provide some immunity.

Jenner, Koch and others then developed vaccines of varying degrees of effectiveness against many of the other major communicable diseases of the time – cholera, tuberculosis, tetanus, diphtheria and rabies.

The germ theory is entrenched, but in later years diseases such as cancer, diabetes and even multiple sclerosis are examined.

Charles Darwin had died in 1802.

Has the 'gene theory' overtaken the 'germ theory'?

c1881   Walter Rudolf Hess (Swiss physiologist) develops the technique of using small electrodes to stimulate specific regions of the brain. Working with dogs and cats he identifies various regions in the brain.

c1882   Paul Ehrlich introduces his diazo reaction for diagnosing typhoid fever.

Robert Koch discovers the bacterium that causes tuberculosis, the first definite association of a germ with a specific human disease.

Joseph Breuer (Viennese physician) uses hypnosis to treat hysteria. It is the beginning of psychoanalysis.

c1883 Francis Galton's 'Enquiries into Human Faculty' introduces the term eugenics, and suggests that human beings can be improved by selective breeding.

Edwin Klebs and Friedrich Lofflet identify the diphtheria bacillus.

Robert Koch discovers Cholera vibrio, the bacterium that causes cholera, and shows that cholera can be transmitted by food and drinking water.

Sir Cyril Lodowic Burt (English psychologist) is born in Stratford-upon-Avon. He founded Mensa, a society for the intellectually gifted. He firmly believes that intelligence is inherited, and makes up data to prove that he is correct.

c1884 Carl Koller (Czech-American surgeon) uses cocaine as a local anaesthetic.

Ilya Illich Mechnikov (Russian-French bacteriologist) discovers phagocytes in the body, mobile white blood cells that attack and devour invading organisms.

Edwin Klebs (German pathologist) isolates the diphtheria bacillus.

Max Tubner (German physiologist) discovers that the body gets energy from carbohydrates, fats and proteins after stripping away nitrogen for other uses.

1885 Louis Pasteur develops a vaccine against hydrophobia (rabies) and uses it to save the life of a young boy, Joseph Meister, bitten by a rabid dog.

1886 Ernst von Zergmann uses steam to sterilise surgical instruments.

The Pasteur Institute, Paris, is founded.

c1886 Baron Richard von Krafft-Ebing (German neurologist) publishes 'Psychopathia Sexualis' (Sexual Psychopathy). It is the first account of abnormal sexual practices in humans and introduces such terms as paranoia, sadism and masochism.

1887 Phenacetin is discovered.

c1887 Louis J. Girard (Baylor College of Medicine in Houston, Texas) develops the first form of contact lens. It covers the whites of the eye as well as the cornea.

Wolfgang Kohler (Russian-German-American psychologist) is one of the founders of the Gestalt school of psychology. Best known for his experiments with chimpanzees in order to demonstrate their problem-solving ability.

Bernardo Alberto Houssay, (Argentinian physiologist) demonstrates that the pituitary gland produces a hormone that has the opposite effect of insulin, showing the complexity of the endocrine system.

c1889 Von Mehring and Minkowski prove that the pancreas secretes insulin, preventing diabetes.

c1890 Joseph Lister demonstrates antiseptic surgery.

William Halsted (American surgeon) introduces the practice of wearing sterilised rubber gloves during surgery.

c1892 The American Psychological Association is founded.

Theobald Smith (American pathologist) discovers that Texas cattle fever is spread by ticks. This is the first known arthropod vector for disease and paves the way for the discovery of how such diseases as malaria, typhus and Lyme disease are spread.

c1893 William Osler (English-American-Canadian physician) publishes 'The Principles and Practice of Medicine', which becomes a standard textbook in the United States.

Daniel Williams (American surgeon) performs the first open-heart surgery on a patient injured by a knife wound.

Sigmund Freud's and Josef Breuer's collaboration in studying the psychic mechanism of hysterical phenomena becomes the foundation of psychoanalysis.

c1898 Paul-Louis Simond, fighting the bubonic plague pandemic in Bombay, realises that fleas on rats transmit the disease to humans.

DON'T FEEL GUILTY....!

Henry Havelock Ellis (1859-1939), English physician and writer on sex, was the son of a sea captain.

He travelled widely before studying medicine at St. Thomas' Hospital in London. He had a number of women followers, including Olive Schreiner, the South African writer feminist. Havelock Ellis caused tremendous controversy with his seven-volume 'Studies in the Psychology of Sex' (1897-1928, revised in 1936)

It was a detached treatment of sex unmarred by any guilt feelings. The books were banned in Britain.

He was the first editor of the Mermaid series of unexpurgated reprints of Elizabethan and Jacobean drama, and also edited the Contemporary Science series.

In 1918 he published 'The Erotic Rights of Women', and his autobiography 'My Life' was published posthumously in 1940.

c1899 Felix Hoffman develops aspirin.

Sigmund Freud founds psychiatry.

c1900 Hugo Marie de Vries (Netherlands), Karl Franz Joseph Correns (Germany) and Erich Tschermak von Seysenegg (Austria) re-discover, quite independently, Gregor Mendel's work on genetics which had been ignored for 40 years.

Walter Stanborough Sutton (America) states that chromosomes are paired and may be the carriers of heredity. His 'The Chromosomes Theory of Heredity' contains detailed studies that support his proposals: that genes are carried by chromosomes. He argues that each egg or sperm cell contains only one of each chromosome pair, which accounts for the random factor in heredity.

c1900 Karl Landsteiner (Austrian doctor) shows that there are at least three different types of human blood (A, B and O) some of which are incompatible. The serum of a person can agglutinate red globules of a donor from an incompatible group.

c1901 Havelock Ellis starts his 'Studies in the Psychology of Sex'.

Sigmund Freud's 'Zur Psychopathologie des Alltags' (the Psychopathology of Everyday Life) introduces the famous concept of the 'Freudian slip'.

AVOID THAT FREUDIAN SLIP

Beware! You may, without realising it, release your unconscious desires into your conscious discussions with others.

It has been related to disguised manifestations of repressed sexual desires.

That was Freud's theory. Later, he elaborated his theory of the division of the unconscious mind into the 'Id', the 'Ego' and the 'Super-Ego'.

Sigmund Freud (1856-1939) was an Austrian neurologist and studied medicine at Vienna.

He collaborated with Joseph Breuer in the treatment of hysteria, and then studied in Paris under Jean Martin Charcot.

It was then that he changed from neurology (a scientific study of the nerve systems) to the more imaginative study of psychoanalysis.

There followed the development of his ideas with Alfred Adler and Carl Jung.

In 1930 he was awarded the prestigious Goethe prize, and in 1933 he published 'Why War?' in collaboration with Albert Einstein.

Great minds think alike.

---

c1902 Alfred Adler (Astria) joins Freud and others to form the first psychoanalytic society.

Ivan Petrovich Pavlov formulates his law of learning by conditioning. He demonstrates that a dog trained by giving it food at the same time that a bell is rung will soon learn to salivate at the sound of a bell without food being present.

c1903 Willem Einthoven (Dutch physiologist) develops the string galvanometer, the forerunner of the electrocardiograph, used to measure tiny electrical currents produced by the heart.

Gregory Pincus (American biologist) becomes one of the pioneers of the birth-control pill.

c1904 W.C. Gorgas eradicates yellow fever in Panama Canal zone.

c1905 Alfred Binet (France), V.Henri and T.Simon develop the intelligence test.

1905   Alexis Carrel (France) working at the Rockefeller Institute in New York City, develops techniques for severed blood vessels, paving the way for organ transplantation.

George Washington Crile performs the first direct blood transfusion.

J.B.Murphy develops the first artificial joints for use in the hip of an arthritic patient.

c1906   The term 'allergy' is introduced by Clemens von Pirquet.

The United States Food and Drugs Act is enacted.

China and Britain agree to a reduction in opium production.

c1909   T.H.Morgan begins researches in genetics.

Wilhelm Johannsen (Denmark) coins the following terms:

'gene' to describe the carrier of heredity

'genotype' to describe the genetic constitution of an organism

'phenotype' to describe the actual organism, which results from a combination of the genotype and various environmental factors.

c1910   Major Frank Woodbury (US Army Medical Corps) introduces the use of tincture of iodine as a disinfectant for wounds.

Paul Ehrlich synthesises the first specific bacterial agent, salversan. It is a cure for syphilis.

c1911   William Hill (English doctor) develops the first gastroscope, a tube that can be swallowed by a patient so that the doctor may look at the inside of a patient's stomach through the tube.

c1912   Casimir Funk (Polish-American biochemist) coins the term 'vitamin' for a class of substances that Frederick Hopkins had found to be important to health, and which had previously been called accessory food factors.

Paul Ehrlich introduces acriflavine as antiseptic.

c1913   John Jacob Abel (America) develops the first artificial kidney.

Frank Mallory discovers the bacterium causing whooping cough.

A. Salomen (German surgeon) develops mammography for diagnosing breast cancer.

Bela Schick introduces the Schick test for diphtheria.

c1914   Dr. Alexis Carrel performs the first successful heart surgery on a dog.

c1915   Joseph Goldberger (Austrian-American physician) establishes that a vitamin deficiency causes pellagra.

c1915   There are tetanus epidemics in the trenches. It's World War I, of course.

Margaret Sanger is jailed for writing 'Family Limitation', the first book on birth control.

c1916   Sympathectomy for relief of angina pectoris is performed for the first time by Ionescu.

Blood for transfusion is refrigerated.

c1916   Margaret Sanger joins in opening the first birth control clinic.

c1917   Carl Gustav Jung (Switzerland) 'Psychology of the Unconscious' is published

c1917   Wagner von Jauregg (Austria) treats syphilitic paralysis by injecting malaria.

c1920 Harvey Cushing (American surgeon) develops new techniques in brain surgery.

c1921 Alexander Fleming (Scotland) discovers the antibacterial substance Lysozyme in saliva, mucus, and tears. A fortuitous accident is involved. He has a cold and some of his mucus drips onto a culture plate where it dissolves the bacteria which is present.

THE GREAT FLEMING

No, not Ian Fleming, but Sir Alexander Fleming (1881-1955) who discovered penicillin in 1928.

Most doctors have a common question – "Are you allergic to penicillin?" It was discovered by a chance exposure in 1928, and because Fleming had insufficient chemical knowledge he had to wait eleven years before two brilliant experimentalists, Howard Florey and Ernst Chain, were able to effect a method of production of that volatile drug.

Fleming shared with them the 1945 Nobel prize for physiology or medicine, and he was appointed professor of bacteriology at London in 1938.

The other Fleming, Ian, was never knighted, nor did he win the Nobel prize. Yet he was responsible for some famous novels in which hundreds of actors 'died'.

Sir Alexander Fleming might have saved them from final extinction with his wonder drug – penicillin!

---

c1921 Ernst Kretschmer's 'Physique and Character' suggests that the mental state of a person is related to his (or her) body build.

T.H.Morgan (American biologist) postulates the chromosome theory of heredity.

c1922 Herbert Mclean Evans and K.J.Scott discover vitamin E.

Insulin is first used to treat diabetes.

Elmer McCollum discovers vitamin D in cod liver oil and uses it for treating rickets.

c1923 Sigmund Freud's 'The Ego and the Id' is published.

The first birth-control clinic is opened in New York.

c1925 George Hoyt Whipple (America) finds that iron is an important constituent of red blood cells.

c1926 Vitamin B in its pure form is isolated by B.C.P.Jansen and W.F.Donath.

W.P.Murphy and George Minot treat pernicious anaemia with liver extract.

c1927 'Conditioned Reflexes' is published by I.P.Pavlov.

Experiments on pernicious anaemia and tuberculosis are conducted by George Whipple.

The Industrial Health and Safety Centre is opened in London.

Paul Drinker and Louis Shaw develop the 'iron lung', a device for mechanical artificial respiration.

c1928 Alexander Fleming discovers penicillin in moulds. In the 1940s its clinical use in therapy starts. Howard Florey and Ernst Chain develop it further and it is learned how to manufacture it in quantity.

c1929 Manfred J.Sankel introduces insulin shock for the treatment of schizophrenia.

c1932 Vitamin D is discovered.

Gerhard Domagk (German bacteriologist and pathologist) begins work on the sulphonamide drugs, a kind of antibiotic.

ECT (Electro-convulsive therapy) is developed.

c1933 Tadeusz Reichstein synthesises pure vitamin C.

Vitamin B_2 (Riboflavin) is recognised by R.Kuhn, Szent-Gyorgi and Wagner von Jauregg.

c1934 Adolph Butenandt isolates the first crystalline male hormone – androsterone.

c1935 Leopold Ruzicka (Yugoslavian chemist) finds the structure of testosterone, a male sex hormone.

c1936 Andrei Nikolaevitch Belozersky isolates DNA in the pure state for the first time.

Dr. Alexis Carrel develops an artificial heart.

c1937 Conrad Arnold Elvehjem discovers vitamin A.

c1938 Vitamin E is chemically identified by Karter, Salomon and Fritzsche.

c1939 Edward Adelbert Doisy (America) isolates Vitamin K.

c1940 Penicillin is developed as a practical antibiotic by Howard Florey.

c1941 Selman Abraham Waksman (Russian-American microbiologist) coins the term 'antibiotic' to describe substances that kill bacteria without injuring other forms of life.

c1943 Penicillin is successfully used in the treatment of chronic diseases.

Wilhelm Kolff (Dutch doctor) develops the first kidney dialysis machine.

c1944 Alfred Blalock performs the first 'blue baby' operation, correcting blood supply to the lungs of a female infant.

Oswald Theodore Avery, Colin MacLeod and Maclyn McCarthy determine that deoxyribonucleic acid (DNA) is the hereditary material for almost all living materials.

THE 'DNA' PHENOMENON

Did those great physicians and surgeons, from Imhotep to the present, wonder at creation?

Did they stare at the skies, searching for a message from above; a message that would explain to them the mystery of life?

Darwin's 'Origin of the Species' created a great furore and is still a subject for considerable discussion.

Francis Crick, born in 1916, with his American colleague, James Dewey Watson, brought real consternation to the world with his construction at the Cavendish Laboratory, Cambridge, of the structure of DNA.

It was a molecular model of the complex genetic material deoxyribonucleic acid (DNA).

This has led to far-reaching discoveries concerning the genetic code.

With Watson and Maurice H.Wilkins he was awarded the Nobel prize for medicine and physiology in 1962.

What a great discovery!

---

c1945 The Nobel Prize for Physiology or Medicine is awarded to Sir Alexander Fleming, Sir Howard W.Florey and Ernst Boris Chain. It is for their discovery of penicillin and research into its value as a weapon against infectious disease.

c1948 The first World Health Assembly meets in Geneva.

c1949 Cortisone is discovered by Philip Hench.

c1950 Antihistamines become popular remedy for colds and allergies.

c1951 A heart-lung machine for heart operations is devised by J.Andre-Thomas.

John Gibbon (an American surgeon) develops the heart-lung machine.

c1952 Robert Wallace Wilkins discovers that reserpine is a tranquiliser, the first one found. He had been using it to treat high blood pressure.

A polio epidemic in the United States affects 47,665 persons.

Douglas Bevis (English doctor) develops amniocentesis, a method of examining the genetic heritage of a foetus while it is still in the womb.

The world's first sex-change operation is performed on George Jorgensen, who becomes known to the world as Christine.

Jonas Edward Salk (America) develops a killed-virus vaccine against polio. It is used for mass inoculations starting in 1954 and successfully prevents the disease. Later it is superseded by a live-virus vaccine developed by Albert Sabin.

THE SALK VACCINE

Jonas Edward Salk was born in 1914, the son of a garment worker in New York City.

He taught medicine at the New York University College of Medicine and at several other schools of medicine.

In 1963 he became director of the Salk Institute in San Diego, California.

By the time he moved to California he was known world-wide for his work on the Salk Vaccine against poliomyelitis.

c1952 Jean Dausset (France) discovers that people who have had repeated blood transfusions eventually develop antibodies to the blood being transfused, an observation later used in typing tissue for organ transplants.

c1953 Evarts A.Graham and Ernest L.Wydner demonstrate that tars from tobacco smoke cause cancer in mice.

Alfred C.Kinsey publishes 'Sexual Behaviour in the Human Female'.

Lung cancer is reported attributable to cigarette smoking.

Rosalind Elsie Franklin (Britain) and Maurice Hugh Frederick Williams (British physicist) make X-ray studies of deoxyribonucleic acid (DNA) that allow James Watson and Francis Crick to determine its structure.

James Dewey Watson (America) and Francis H.Crick (Britain) develop the model for DNA, explaining how the giant molecule is capable of transmitting heredity in living organisms.

c1953   John H.Gibbon, Jr., uses his heart-lung machine to keep Cecelia Bavolek alive while operating successfully on her heart, the first use of the machine on a human being.

Frederick Sanger (England) becomes the first to determine the structure of the protein – insulin.

c1954   Chloropromazine (Thorazine) is introduced for the treatment of mental disorders.

c1955   Sir Edward Mellanby (England) dies. His work with vitamin A paved the way for the discovery of vitamin D.

Dorothy Hodgkin discovers a liver extract for treating pernicious anaemia (vitamin B_{12}).

c1956   Oral vaccine is developed by Albert Sabin against polio.

c1957   Giberellin, a growth-producing hormone, is isolated.

The high-speed, painless dental drill is developed in the United States.

c1958   Bifocal contact lenses are introduced.

c1960   American Heart Association issues a report attributing higher death rates among middle-aged men to heavy smoking of cigarettes.

c1961   Frank L.Horsfall, Jr., announces that all forms of cancer result from changes in the DNA of cells.

c1962   Lasers are used in eye surgery for the first time.

c1963   Dr. Michael De Bakey (America) first uses an artificial heart to take over the circulation of a patient's blood during heart surgery.

c1964   Home kidney dialysis is introduced in the UK and the USA.

Baruch S. Blumberg (America) discovers the 'Australian antigen', which is the key to the development of a vaccine for hepatitis B.

c1965   A vaccine against measles becomes available.

Soft contact lenses are invented.

Harry Harlow demonstrates that monkeys reared in total isolation show great emotional impairment for the rest of their lives!

c1966   The French Academy of Medicine is the first medical group to use brain inactivity instead of heart stoppage as the clinical definition of death.

Konrad Lorenz's 'On Aggression' argues that only human beings intentionally kill members of their own species.

c1967   Clomiphene is introduced to increase fertility. It results in an increase in multiple births.

Mammography for detecting breast cancer is introduced.

c1967   Dr. Irving S.Cooper (America) develops cryosurgery as a means of treating Parkinson's disease.

'The Naked Ape' by Desmond Morris is published.

A 20-year study of fluoridation shows that dental cavities have been reduced by 58% as a result of adding fluorides to the water supply.

Christiaan Neelthing Barnard (South African surgeon) performs the first partially successful human heart transplant. Louis Washkansky is the recipient of the new heart and lives for 18 days.

Rene Favaloro (American surgeon) develops the coronary bypass operation.

c1968 Christiaan Barnard performs a second human heart transplant. The patient, Philip Blaiberg, lives for 74 days with his new heart.

c1969 Denton Cooley and Domingo Liotta (America) replace the diseased heart of Haskell Karp with the first artificial heart to be used in a human being. The patient lives for 3 days.

c1974 Genetic engineering, in which the genes of one organism are inserted in another, is viewed with alarm by a committee of 139 scientists from the US National Academy of Sciences and 18 other nations led by Paul Berg (America). The committee calls for a halt in specified research until the implications are better understood.

c1976 The viral cause of multiple sclerosis is discovered.

1978 The first human baby conceived outside the body – called a test-tube baby – is born to Lesley Brown in the United Kingdom.

c1980 A team headed by Martin Cline succeeds in transferring a gene from one mouse to another and having the gene function.

The World Health Organisation declares that smallpox is eradicated!

c1981 Chinese scientists become the first to clone successfully a fish – a golden carp!

The US Centres for Disease Control recognises acquired immune deficiency syndrome (AIDS) for the first time.

The genetic code for the hepatitis B surface antigen is found, opening up the possibility of a bio-engineered vaccine.

c1984 The American Heart Association lists smoking as a risk factor for strokes for the first time.

A vaccine for leprosy is developed.

William H.Clewall (American surgeon) performs the first successful surgery on a foetus before birth.

c1984 Alec Jeffreys discovers the technique of genetic fingerprinting, the identification of certain core sequences of DNA unique to each person. This method can not only be used for identifiying individuals but also for establishing family relationships.

c1985 Lasers are used in the USA for the first time to clean out clogged arteries.

c1987 David C. Page and his colleagues announce their discovery of the gene that initiates maleness in mammals. It appears to be a single gene on the Y chromosome that starts the sequence that leads to the development of testes instead of ovaries.

c1988 Graham Colditz and a team of co-workers announce that a study of 120,000 nurses reveals that women who smoke half a pack of cigarettes a day are twice as likely to have strokes as non-smokers, while women who smoke two packs a day are six times as likely.

GENETIC ENGINEERING

The path toward genetic engineering was opened in 1952 when Joshua Lederberg discovered that bacteria, like some protists, conjugate to exchange genetic material.

It led him to perceive that there are two populations of bacteria, which he called M and F.

The next year William Hayes established that the plasmid consists of genetic material.

By then it was clear that genes were DNA.

In 1959 Japanese scientists discovered that the genes for drug resistance were carried on plasmids, and therefore were carried around from bacterium to bacterium.

There had been another line of research.

Immediately after World War II, a number of biologists made an intensive study of viruses that infect bacteria, which are collectively called bacteriophages, or just phages.

The research demonstrated that genes are DNA and not protein.

In 1946 Max Delbruck and Alfred Hershey independently showed that the gene from phages could spontaneously combine.

Werner Arber studied the mutation process in phages in detail, and discovered that bacteria resist phages by splitting the phage DNA with enzymes.

In 1969, Jonathan Beckwith and his co-workers became the first to isolate a single gene.

It was a bacterial gene for a part of the metabolism of sugar.

In 1973 Stanley H. Cohen and Herbert W. Brown combined the restriction enzymes with plasmids with isolation of specific genes to introduce genetic engineering.

But not all scientists thought that this was a good thing, and in July 1974, Paul Berg and other biologists met under the auspices of the US National Academy of Sciences to draw up guidelines that would prohibit certain kinds of genetic engineering.

Some of the techniques used in genetic engineering have made it possible to find markers for a number of diseases.

Other techniques indicate an interference with natural growth, a philosophical problem which humankind has to deal with.

Animals and plants can hardly be expected to have a say in that final decision.

Perhaps George Orwell has the answer?

WHAT ON EARTH IS A GENETIC MARKER?

Or, put another way, what on another planet could be a genetic marker?

There are approximately 3,000 human diseases which are now known to be caused by genes.

A person who inherits a single gene for Huntingdon's disease, or two genes for cystic fibrosis, could have that disease.

The problem is that there could be as many as 2,000,000 of them for any given person.

Locating which gene is involved in a particular disease is not too easy.

And that, dear reader, is very much an under-statement!

Edward M.Southern developed a method to pick out specific pieces of DNA, called Southern blotting.

Suppose you know that a certain genetic disease occurs in your family. You won't know which gene is involved, but you know which members of the family are affected.

There could be an identifiable piece of DNA from affected or unaffected family members. That gives the clue to the marker for the gene.

By suitable separation and testing of different chromosomes a scientist can use the marker to locate the chromosome on which the suspect gene can be found.

Kay Davies and Robert Williamson used these methods to locate the first marker for Duchenne muscular dystrophy.

Identifying genetic markers requires a careful study of a large family, as different families may have different markers for the same gene.

Mapping all the useful genetic markers on each chromosome will help to cut short the effort to locate specific genes.

In 1988 the US National Academy of Sciences called for a major national effort to map the genes of human beings.

X-rays are often shown to patients to indicate where physical problems exist in the body.

When will you be shown a map of your personal genome (a totality of all your own genes) so that you can recognise your personal medical problem?

And, if you intend to relocate yourself on another planet, which of your personal genes will you select in order to survive on your chosen planet?

The choice will be yours!

SOME OF THE VOLUNTARY ORGANISATIONS WHICH SUPPORT SUFFERERS OF VARIOUS MEDICAL CONDITIONS IN THIS POCKET REFERENCE BOOK

Alcohol Concern – 305 Grays Inn Road, London WC1X 8QF. 0171 833 3471.

Alcohol – Scottish Council on – 137-145 Sauchiehall Street, Glasgow G2 3EW. 0141 333 9677.

Alcoholics Anonymous – PO Box 1, Stonebow House, Stonebow, York Y01 2NT. 01904 644026/7/8/9

Alzheimer's Disease Society – Gordon House, 10 Greenwood Place, London SW1P 1PH. 0171 306 0606

Ankylosing Spondylitis – The National Association for – 5 Grosvenor Crescent, London SW1X 7EI. 0171 235 9585.

Anorexics Anonymous – 24 Westmoreland Place, London SW13 9RY. 0181 748 3994.

Arthritis and Rheumatism Council for Research – PO Box 177, Chesterfield, Derbyshire S41 7QT. 01246 558033.

Asthma – National Campaign – Providence House, Providence Place, London N1 0NT. 0171 226 2240.

Autistic – The National Society – 276 Willesden Road, London NW2 5RB. 0181 451 1114.

Back Pain – The National Association – Grundy House, 31–33 Park Road, Teddington, Middlesex. TW11 OAB. 0171 977 5474.

Blind – Royal National Institute for the – 224 Great Portland Street, London W1N 6AA. 0171 388 1266.

Colitis and Crohn's Disease – The National Association for – 98a London Road, St Albans, Hertfordshire AL1 1NX. 01727 44296.

Colostomy – British Association – 15 Station Road, Reading, Berks RG1 1LG. 01734 391537

Cystic Fibrosis Research Trust – Alexandra House, 5 Blyth Road, Bromley, Kent BR1 3RS. 0181 464 7211.

Diabetic – British Association – 10 Queen Anne Street, London W1M OBD. 0171 323 1531.

Down's Syndrome Association – 155 Mitcham Road, London SW17 9PG. 0181 682 4001.

Dyslexia – British Association – 98 Reading Road, Reading, Berks RG1 5AU. 01734 662677.

Eating Disorders Association – Sackville Place, 44 Magdalen Street, Norwich NR3 1JE. 01603 621414.

Epilepsy Association of Scotland – 48 Govan Road, Glasgow G51 1JL. 0141 427 4911.

Epilepsy – British Association – Anstey House, 40 Hanover Square, Leeds, LS3 1BE. 01532 439393.

Gender Dysphoric Trust International – BM Box No.7624 , London WC1N 3XN. 01323 641100.

Huntingdon's Disease Association – 108 Battersea High Street, London SW11 9PG. 0171 223 700

Ileostomy Association of Great Britain and Ireland – Amblehurst House, Black Scotch Lane, Mansfield, Notts NG18 4PF. 01623 28099.

Infant Deaths – Foundation for the Study of – 35 Belgrave Square, London. SW1X 8QB. 0171 235 0965.

Kidney Research Fund – National – 3 Archers Court, Stukeley Road, Huntingdon, Cambs PE18 6XG. 01480 454828.

Mental Health Foundation – 37 Mortimer Street, London W1N 7RG. 0171 580 0141.

Mental Health (MIND) – National Association for – 22 Harley Street, London W1N 2ED. 0171 637 0741.

Mentally Handicapped Children and Adults (Mencap) – The Royal Society for – 123 Golden Lane, London EC1Y ORT. 0171 454 0454.

Mentally Handicapped – The Scottish Society for – Belmbank Street, Glasgow G2 4QA. 0141 226 4541.

Motor Neurone Association – PO Box 246, Northampton, NN1 2PP. 01604 25050, 22269.

Multiple Sclerosis Society of Great Britain & Northern Ireland – 25 Effie Road, London SW6 1EE. 0181 736 6267.

Muscular Dystrophy Group of Great Britain – The – 7 - 11 Prescott Place, London SW4 6BT. 0171 720 8055.

Myaesthenia Gravis Association – Keynes House, 77 Nottingham Road, Derby DE1 3QS. 01332 290219.

Osteoporosis Society – The National – PO Box 10, Radstock, Bath BA3 3YB. 01761 432472.

Parkinson's Disease Society of Great Britain – 22 Upper Woburn Place, London WC1H ORA. 0171 383 3513.

Phobics Society – The – 4 Cheltenham Road, Chorlton Cum Hardy, Manchester M21 1QW. 0161 881 1937.

Schizophrenia Fellowship – National – London Advisory Centre – 197 Kings Cross Road, London. WC1X 9DB. 0171 837 6436.

Scope – 12 Park Crescent, London W1N 4EQ. 0171 636 5020.

Sickle Cell Society – The – Green Lodge, 54 Station Road, London. NW10 4UA. 0181 961 7795/40

Spastics – The Scottish Council for – 22 Corstorhine Road, Edinburgh,EH12 6HP. 0131 337 987

Spina Bifida and Hydrocephalus – The Association for – Asbah House, 42 Park Road, Peterborough PE1 20Q. 01733 555988.

Spina Bifida Association – The Scottish – 190 Queensferry Road, Edinburgh EH4 2BW. 0131 332 0743.

Spinal Injuries Association – Newpoint House, 76 St James Lane, Muswell Hill,London N10 3DF. 0181 444 2121.

Transexuals – Partners Group for Partners and Families of – BM Box 6093, London WC1N 3XX. 01373 641100.

Tuberous Sclerosis Association of Great Britain – Little Barnsley Farm, Catshill, Bromsgrove, Worcs B61 ONQ. 01527 71828.